THE LAST
HALLOWEEN

By
Peter Christian Olsen

Table of Contents

Introduction

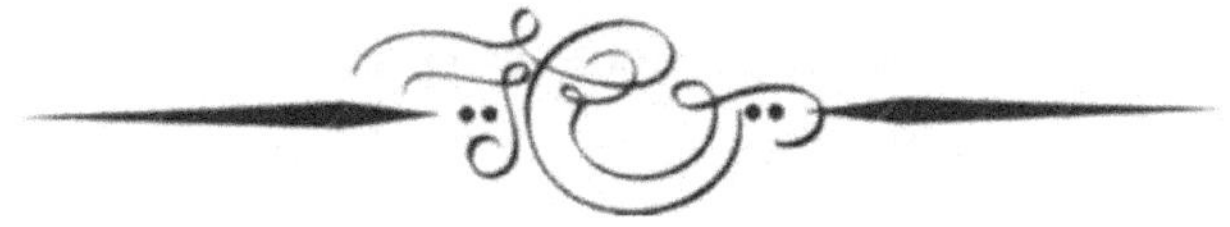

The life of the dead is placed

In the memory of the living

- Marcos Tullius Cicero

Tragedy occurs in human lives so that we will learn
to reach out and comfort others.

- C.S.Lewis

The greatest tragedy in life is not death; instead, it is living life without purpose. This concept promoted by Myles Munroe is profoundly perceptive, profound because it captures an aspect of life not customarily understood, perceptive because it's a truth we often ignore. The emotional response to the loss of a loved one can be overwhelming, and Grief is hard work. We know from experience that grieving can be an agonizing experience. It takes effort and time to get past the grief.

The immediate and customary reaction to death is a profound loss, the experience of ultimate defeat, the point of no return. Despite any philosophical or theological discernment about death, the emotional reaction usually takes priority. Feelings of despondency and hopelessness become ingrained and can hang around for months or even years. It is never easy to just move on despite the encouragement we get from friends. Death can be tragic I learned that from personal experience.

When tragedy occurs in one set of circumstances, however, that tragedy can be the impulse that sets in motion a whole new set of circumstances.

Sometimes change happens spontaneously, unplanned, and without forethought or prediction. Circumstances change, demanding new insights and new experiences. Change has happened to me.

This book serves two purposes; it meanders down two separate pathways, two separated journeys; each linked to the other. First of all, it is a narrative about the last few months of my wife's life. It's not so much about her; rather, her experience is the context in which I write about myself and my response to her last days. She might deserve to be central to the story but if truth be told, it's my story, my experience, my responses, my feelings, and my actions that are central to my narrative.

Secondly, I then share some insight about death and dying that emulates from my personal experience of being a hospice chaplain. A hospice chaplain's primary focus is to provide spiritual care to those suffering from a terminal illness. Such care, of course, also extends to their families. Interspersed throughout the book are various scenarios and patient stories of my hospice chaplains' experiences.

So how are these two experiences linked together? How I responded to my wife's death became the impetus for my becoming a hospice chaplain—sort of a redemptive activity. Because I felt so inept at caretaking for my wife, I sought redemption in my ability and experience of being a chaplain to hospice patients.

This narrative does not follow a chronological order. The exception to this statement is that the course of "Ariel's Stories" follows events in the order of their occurrence. In between these events, I share narratives of my experience of being a hospice chaplain. Please note: I became a hospice chaplain after Ariel's death, not during her dying.

Chapter 1

The Last Halloween

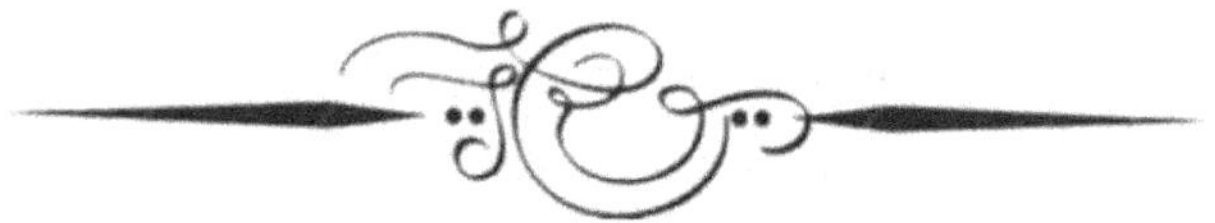

When you are joyous, look deep into your heart and you shall find it is only that which has given you sorrow that is giving you joy. When you are sorrowful look again in your heart, and you shall see that in truth you are weeping for that which has been your delight.

- Khalil Gibran

"I think this will be my last Halloween," she told me. My wife Ariel and I were sitting on the living room couch watching the evening news. Our kids were grown and out of the house with families of their own. Ariel and I discovered we could now spend time together unencumbered by the needs of children. We were beginning to enjoy our time alone together; a time for retirement and rediscover.

I had already retired from my full-time position in ministry and bided my time until Ariel reached her retirement status. We anticipated spending retirement time together, but so far without specific goals. Despite our previous conversations about retirement, I had uncertainties about Ariel's intentions. Ariel focused on her nursing, a career she chose from the age of twelve and from which she never wavered in her enthusiasm. I thought it might be too difficult for her to withdraw. Instead, I had a hunch she was considering part-time work after retirement.

Much of our time together was reflective, a time when we consciously shared anything new that occurred each day, what we were feeling, plans for the next day, if there were any, and other concerns we thought imperative but not overly important. We often talked about our grandchildren. Grandchildren had taken on a strong priority in our lives.

This evening Ariel focused on putting food away while I washed the few dishes we used. We completed these chores by six-thirty in time to watch the evening news. I sat on the living room couch and turned on the news. Ariel remained in the kitchen. That's when she suddenly exclaimed without prompting, "I need to talk with you."

The tone of her voice caught me by surprise. We rarely used this time to engage in serious conversation; so, when she exclaimed with emphasis, "I NEED" to talk with you," I was instantly aware that something important was on her mind. "I need to talk," I surmised as a clue to something imperative. I put the television on pause and directed my attention toward her.

"Yeah, what's up?" I asked her.

She didn't immediately respond. Her hesitation allowed me a moment to refocus on the news.

"Peter, pay attention," She reiterated her thoughts. "Peter, I need to tell you something, and I don't want you to get upset." She said this with an inflection I interpreted as "you had better listen up and take heed." When she had something important to share, she became focused, requiring my full responsiveness.

"Okay," I said, facing her directly. "I'll try not to get upset, but that depends on what you tell me." I had no clue what was bothering her. Her facial expression, however, gave her away. She was upset. Instead of looking directly at me as she normally did when we spoke together, her eyes randomly wandered around the room. I couldn't recall any pressing issues between us that needed attention, at least not at that moment, so I remained puzzled and wondered what might be on her mind. She remained standing in the kitchen doorway. She came and stood close by me.

She took a deep breath. "Halloween is my favorite holiday," she stated. "I don't know why; it just is, but I am scared that this might be my last Halloween. Something strange is happening to my body."

"Oh my God," I replied. I sounded surprised, but not entirely. Her declaration was something I was already aware of as she had casually mentioned before that her back was bothering her. It conjured up all the anxieties I was already feeling but suppressing. I knew she had backaches for which we had not yet found any reason. She continued hurting and found no relief from her pain. I felt her words came as a premonition of what was to come.

She continued. "Something strange is happening, and I am not sure I understand, but I have this feeling this might be my last Halloween." She spoke in such a casual manner, stoically, almost as if she were talking about another person or repeating something she heard about another person, not herself. She then sat down on the couch next to me.

"It feels like my bones are rubbing together, and my muscles are on fire," she told me when I asked how she was feeling. Ariel was always frank and open to me in all our conversations. We shared feelings and didn't shy away from difficult discussions. The one exception was that Ariel hesitated to burden me with personal problems. When something truly bothered her or caused great concern, she hesitated to tell me. She didn't want to upset me unless necessary. She was not a complainer. She did not whine—just the opposite. In forty years of marriage, I can honestly state that I never, and I mean never, heard her reference a derogatory word against another person or utter a complaint. She was always open and honest and positive, and respectful. Her mojo was her magical power never to offend another person.

This day, however, she was bothered, and she wanted me to know. She blurted out her feelings. "I feel shity all over", she exclaimed. She went on to further describe in some detail the frustrations she was feeling about the pain in her back, the symptom of her impending death, a death for which she was unprepared and not expecting. Both Ariel and I looked forward to our future together. Was that now to be by-passed?

I sat still. I looked directly at her. I felt devastated as if I had been punched in my stomach. I gaged and thought I would throw up. It was a knee-jerk reaction, extremely upsetting. How could she so blatantly speak about her impending death so stoically? She was telling me that she was going to die soon with the same demeanor as if telling me she was going to visit her brother.

She began to cry. I choked up. I felt a knot forming in my stomach. I tried to hold back tears. Soon both of us were wiping away a torrent of tears. For a moment, neither of us could garner conversation. We both felt dumbfounded. I reached across the couch and held her tightly, so tightly that I thought she might not be able to breathe. I relinquished my stranglehold, and we both sat quietly on the couch while holding hands, not speaking. After many minutes of agonizing silence, I asked her "What do we do now?"

"I don't know, "she said. "I don't know."

Within three months of our conversation that evening, Ariel was dead.

What happened? We were never sure, never positive, but supposedly she contracted cancer. Cancer did her in. Only after her passing did we find out any diagnosis, and even then, it was not absolute. Tests indicated she had bladder cancer but remain to this day inconclusive.

It took three months for Ariel to eventually succumbed to the ailment. Our first recollection was the onset of some back pains that began following a trip to Disney World with our grandchildren, a simple backache we dismissed as unimportant and insignificant. It initially demanded little attention. Who thinks that back pain could be a precursor foreshadowing doom and death?

We just don't know what life will throw at us. We too easily and haphazardly assume our invincibility and immortality only to recognize too late how shortsighted we had become. We are all terminally ill

Chapter 2

Disney World – Prelude to Destiny

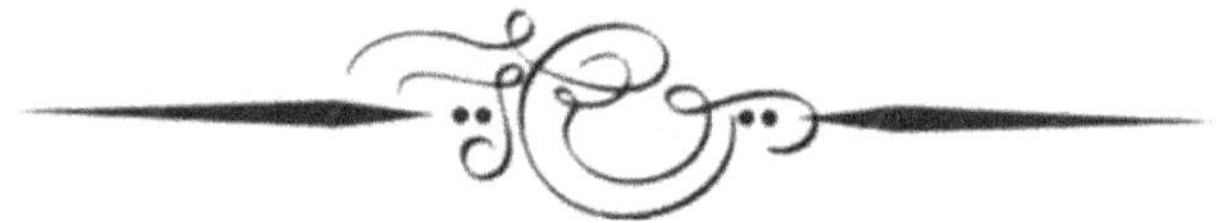

The simplest toy, one which even the youngest child can operate, is called a grandparent.

- Sam Levenson

"Grandpa, can you take us to see Mickey Mouse," my oldest granddaughter asked one day. I suspect it was not spontaneous. She had been thinking about it for most of her short life – all eight years of it. There were times when we were together watching a Disney movie, and an ad appeared advertising Disney World in all its grandeur and color, and Marie would exclaim,

"Can we go there, Grandpa?"

"What do you mean, there?" I asked her.

"To Disney land," she responded.

She succeeded in convincing her younger sister as well, for as soon as Marie stated her request to go visit Mickey, Sophia, five years younger, piped in, "I wanna go too, Grandpa." I don't think she had any concept of Disney World. She habitually imitated her sister.

How could we resist? Grandchildren instinctively know how to wrap grandparents around their little fingers. After consultation with their parents, who reveled in the idea of "missing" their kids for a few days, plans were made for Grandpa and Grandma to take both grandchildren to Disney World in June, immediately after school was dismissed for the summer. Their parents immediately booked a weekend for themselves alone at the Texas coast. "Don't be in a hurry to get back," they told us.

June is not the optimal time to visit Florida. Unfortunately, Disney World is in Florida. It gets hot in June, miserably hot. The heat combined with the humidity becomes unbearable. Since school is out, the crowds are incredibly huge. It appeared as if every child between the ages of two and ten planned to be present, along with either Mom and Dad or Grandpa and Grandma or both. Because of work schedules and school attendance issues, we had little choice of time. June was mandatory, only one degree better than July or August.

We arrived enthusiastically, imagining this to be a wonderful, stress-free vacation with the grandchildren, a time of family bonding with memories made to last a lifetime. Not so. Crowds completely engulfed us while at the park. Lines for rides were unimaginably long, and wait times exceeded ninety minutes. The temperature reached the upper nineties. Grandpa suffered from heatstroke while buckets full of perspiration dripped off his chin. Grandma tried to smile but gritted her teeth and suffered through the days. The kids, however, loved every minute.

Rather than staying in the park, we booked a hotel nearby that had a swimming pool. We convinced the kids it was part of the park. We slept together in one room. When exhausted by the park routine, we escaped to the retail market at Disney World. Fewer people but just as exciting for the kids. Souvenirs galore – plastic alligators, a stuffed Minnie mouse, cherry popsicles, and cotton candy; enough to last their lifetime.

To see the park entirely, much walking is necessary. The youngest granddaughter, Sophia, found it challenging to keep up. She fell behind as we strolled from one attraction to the next, only to stand in line forever before our turn came due. She was so small; we often could not see her in the crowds. Ariel decided it best that she should carry her. Sophie obliged. For the better part of each day, Ariel or I carried Sophia around Disney World, only stopping when our turn arose to ride an attraction, or the necessity arose to stop for a drink or visit a bathroom.

Disney World borders on paradise for young children. It encourages their imaginations to run rampant with all the fairy tale characters like Mickey and Minnie and Goofy and Cinderella and the seven dwarfs constantly available. The grandchildren's eyes looked like saucers as they focused on all the imaginary characters that suddenly appeared real to them.

For an adult (referring to me), I could not imagine Disney World as a pleasant place. Don't get me wrong. I enjoyed the excitement the kids experienced just walking through the park and viewing all the enchanted places. The wide-eyed stares, the anticipation of riding in "It's A Small World," having pictures taken with Ariel, the mermaid, is true magic for the kids. Their excitement was my delight.

But too much "delight" can cause fatigue. If left to my own devices, I would choose a root canal before a trip to Disney World. I do have adult friends who cherished their time at the park, but as of this writing, most of them are experiencing some dementia. I cannot comprehend how such torture can be fulfilling for an adult. It has got to be a labor of love, love for the grandchildren. I felt like the original suffering servant, destined for torture for the sake of pleasing the kids.

I must admit that I went reluctantly and hesitated ever to go again, but I would not have canceled this trip for all the money in the world. To see the delight on our grandchildren's faces and hear their happy chatter made the whole experience meaningful, something not to be squandered.

The excursion to Disney World proved to be a highlight of our time with the grandchildren. Ariel and I, despite the challenges of the park - the weather, the crowds, the lines, and the costs- felt we had mentally logged a memory that would bring joy to our hearts for many years. Neither of us knew, clearly not our kids or the grandchildren, that Grandma would be dead in four months. I feel assured that her memory with the grandchildren only died ten minutes after she did.

Following the Disney family adventure, life for Ariel began a downward spiral of severe backaches, stomach cramps, and sleepless nights. During the first weeks following our trip to Disney World, Ariel stated, not complained, but merely acknowledged (She never complained about anything short of dumb things I did) that her back was bothering her.

"What do you mean, bothering you? How does it bother you? Be specific, please," I asked her.

"I get this pain across my lower back," she replied. She swung her left arm behind her back and drew it across toward the front of her stomach. "Right along here," she instructed. "It's a constant ache."

She told me it ached for a good portion of the day and she got little relief from over-the-counter medications. Little attention was given to her assertion, either by me or by her.

"It's probably from carrying Sophia so much when we were at Disney World," I suggested.

"Maybe," she said. "We'll see."

Little did we realize that this was the first stage of an ongoing experience of incredible frustration, agony, and desperation – the frustration of not knowing her diagnosis, the agony of severe pain she suffered, and the desperation of clinging to the wasted efforts at medical procedures. Doctor appointments and medical procedures, all of which proved of no avail, became a regular part of our daily schedule. Unbeknown to us, she had contracted cancer that remained allusive and undetected by some of the best medical personal available. The only clue we had of the seriousness of her condition was her constant pain. The eventual outcome was her death on October 10, 2009. Her death was too early. She was cremated and her ashes were spread at those places that held great meaning to both her and me. That was her wish.

The period following Ariel's death was a time of much reflection for me. Indeed there were friends and family, and coworkers who attempted to offer condolences and the desire to support. Still, the task ahead of me I knew would be one of acceptance of the inevitable and the challenge of learning to move on. My life had to continue. I had my two daughters and two granddaughters who needed my presence and assurance. We remained a family despite the loss of one crucial part. Thus, began my struggle, my search to regain my life. I knew I had to move on. As it turned out, life would take on many twists and turns, some unexpected deviations, and some significant experiences.

Chapter 3

Moving on: Becoming a Hospice Chaplain

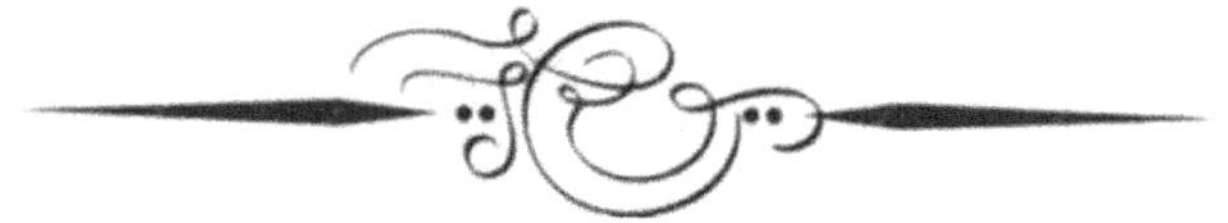

"And once the storm is over, you won't remember how you made it through, how you managed to survive. You won't even be sure, whether the storm is over. But one thing is certain. When you come out of the storm, you won't be the same person who walked in. That's what this storm's all about."

- Haruki Murayama

Before moving on, let me recall for you some lingering thoughts to a time before Ariel's death. Both of us were anticipating retirement. I completed more than thirty years of ministry in various churches and a variety of positions – pastor, educator, counselor, and social activist. She served equal time as a nurse in hospital settings and presently for a hospice program. We liked our vocations, took great pride and satisfaction in what we did for a living, knew that we would miss our working lives, but after many years figured it was time to move on, try something different, and see what else was out there in the world still to be experienced. We realized we were getting older; the kids had left home and were well situated, grandchildren growing like weeds, and family obligations under control. Our health had yet to fail us; both of us exercised regularly, had blood pressure checked, vaccines shots up to date, and diet well monitored.

Travel was foremost on our bucket list. I retired a year and a half previously, and Ariel planned the same thing in less than a year. We shared ideas about where we wanted to go, things we wanted to see, experiences we anticipated in retirement. Even though I suspected retirement would be difficult for Ariel, she still shared eagerly in our future planning. Unfortunately, all was in vain. Three months later, she was dead.

After her death, it was not an easy transition for me; rather, it was a struggle to move on. Many memories, good times, tough times, in-between times, all part of a long history together. However, I realized there was no backing up, no reliving of the past, only a sense of "where do I go from here?"

To talk about moving on after the death of a person with whom you have so much history can feel like a betrayal; that you are attempting to forget about that person, placing her in the background, and replacing her with new thoughts. Did it mean that her life was of such insignificance that I could merely move on without remorse, that our time together had such little meaning that I ignored it? Nothing could be further from the truth. She was my wife, my best friend, my lover, and her passing from this life to another did little to erase her from my life experience. But I had to let go and move on.

Moving on is inevitable and unavoidable. It has to happen sooner or later. I could choose to spend the remaining days of my life in mourning, thinking solely about my great loss, feeling sorry for myself, focused on idolizing the person now gone, but that neither honors the person who passed nor is healthy for the one who survives. When I encountered persons who idolized their deceased spouses and remained stuck in their past, I felt sorry that they choose to end their futures at that point in their lives. The glorification of the deceased often results in misanthropy. I have had discussions since that time with many hospice patients with whom I work. When queried, the majority say what their wish for the spouse who remains behind after death is that they "move on"; that they find fulfillment in their lives even if that means finding another person with whom to share a new life. None indicated they felt any ill will about the surviving spouse moving on.

In the garden of good and evil

Ariel worked as a hospice nurse until she died. Her tenure was over six years, and she was honored as a most compassionate and competent nurse. One day, shortly after I received her ashes back from the mortuary, I contacted the hospice's founding nurse, a longtime friend, and asked if some of Ariel's ashes could be buried in the garden front of the hospice office. I thought it would be a tribute to her. Ariel enjoyed the people she worked with and fully supported the concept of hospice. Having some of her remains buried on the hospice grounds would forever memorialize her contribution to hospice. Better than a headstone, I thought

"Ariel's heart and soul somehow got caught up in hospice nursing," I told her. "I think she would like it if a part of her remained here in the garden. Can I place some of her ashes here?" I asked.

"Absolutely," was her immediate reply.

"Do we need to check with the Board?" I asked. "Should they know and give me permission?"

"Not necessary, "she fired back almost immediately. "Ariel was so much a part of hospice they would feel honored to have her still be around. If she can't be here in person, let her be here in spirit. Let's just do it and ask questions later."

The next morning, she and I met outside the office and walked to the garden area. I bent down and, with my fingers, dug a small hole at the bases of an Esperanza bush that was glowing with bright yellow and orange flowers. Into the hole, I placed a handful of Ariel's ashes. I started to cry. Grief overwhelmed me. I had to wait a moment before I stood up.

"That feels good, "I told my friend. "She is right where she would like to be."

My friend and I walked back toward the office door. Just before we entered, she paused, grabbed my arm, and looked directly at me. "You know what I am thinking," she said. "I think that maybe you ought to come and work with us at Hope

Hospice. We can always use an extra chaplain. Besides, it would be good for you to get out of the house," she added.

"Thanks," I responded. The invitation took me by surprise. I had not yet given thought to my future or what I might do going forward. "I appreciate your offer, but I need a little time to think about that."

The next day, the psychosocial team supervisor at Hope Hospice called me and asked if I would meet with her. I agreed. My first thoughts were that I would be a volunteer chaplain if asked, occasionally filling in when they needed an extra hand. It never occurred to me to go back to work full time. Retired ministers are not at the top of the list for recruitment in the marketplace.

"No," She said. "We need you to work as much as possible."

"So how much might that be," I asked innocently

"We call it PRN," she told me. "I don't know what PRN stands for, but it means as much as you can do and as often as we need someone."

Denial - The great RV escapade

Taking on a new job was not the primary thought at present. I put off answering the supervisor. I had conditioned myself to think that right now, it might be a good idea to buy that RV I had always dreamed about and take off for the hinterlands. I did not yet convince myself that it was what I truly wanted, but the shock of Ariel's death clouded my mind, and I looked for a diversion from having to face life without her. Fleeing from the problem was an option.

I found an RV for sale and, on a lark, offered to buy it. After a little haggling, we decided on a price, and the RV was mine. What was I thinking? I recalled reading John Steinbach's book, *"Travels with Charlie,"* about his adventures traveling the county in a camper with his dog Charlie who served as a symbolic introduction to people he met along the way. I was intrigued by the possibilities of doing something similar. I had no dog but found a bobblehead Jesus, and I thought it would look nice riding on the dashboard and elicit introductions to people who might be skeptical of strangers in RVs. I placed "Jesus" center on the dashboard

I took the RV for a weekend trip to a nearby State Park for a trial run before launching my anticipated cross-country tour. She (RV's are always female) performed like a champion; air conditioning on a hot night, kitchen appliances just like home, double bed with a soft mattress, plug-in electricity, and running water with shower. It seemed too comfortable to be truly camping.

I left the next morning, and while climbing a slight hill heading home, I noticed that the engine was roaring although I was sliding backward down the hill. An oily smell emanated from the engine. It didn't take any mechanical genius to realize something was significantly wrong with the camper. I backed onto the side of the road and hung my head between my hands as I often do while trying to think deeply.

"What could be wrong," I asked myself. "I just had the engine and transmission checked-out; they passed with flying colors." I could think of no options other than to call for a tow, which eventually got me back to the transmission repair center after a wait of some three hours. Transmission repair is an expensive procedure. The costs to fix everything might require me to mortgage my house again. Although I still had fantasies of traveling, reality took over. I gave up my dreams for RV travel and answered the request to become a Hope Hospice chaplain.

A few weeks following the great RV escapade, Hope hospices staffing welcomed me as a PRN chaplain. PRN meant that I agreed to work as needed, needed when hospice had requests for an additional chaplain, and meaning when I had the time to give. It sounded like the ideal working situation, to be able to work when you want and not to work when you don't. It turns out that hospice needed a working chaplain more often than less often, and I found myself working more often than not.

The Education of a Hospice Chaplain

I was not entirely unprepared for this position. A requirement for graduation from theological seminary many years ago was completing a course in Clinical Pastoral ministry. The program expected each student to spend time "counseling" with patients in a hospital. The school assigned me to Boston City Hospital, a quasi-medical and mental hospital that catered mostly to low-income residents.

A component of the experience was to share counseling episodes with other students under the mentorship of a faculty member. These sharing experiences served as critiques of our performance, a learning experience through "constructive" criticism. Sometimes the criticism turned personal and biting. I recall one of these sharing sessions vividly. The patient assigned to me was terminal and expected to die soon.

Mentor: "So Peter, what did you do with this patient?"

Peter: I talked to him

Mentor: "You talked to him? And tell me what does a student pastor talk to a dying person about?

Peter; (I didn't consider that question before). "Well, mostly, we talked about his family."

Mentor: "Did you talk about God?"

Peter: "No, I don't think so."

Mentor: "What about his religion?"

Peter: "Not so much."

Mentor: "How about the meaning of his life; talk about that?"

Peter: "Sometimes. Maybe a little."

Mentor: "Prayer, did you offer him prayer?"

Peter: "Un…sometimes. But not usually, not really." (I felt this was not going well)

Mentor: "So you just visit him and talk about his family."

Peter: "Well he talks. I listen."

Mentor: "Huh." He leaned back in his chair.

Sometime later, I had to share this verbatim conversation with the entire class. The "constructive criticism" flowed swiftly and thoroughly. The class was unimpressed, to say the least, with my understanding at being insightful and empathetic.

As I read through my responses, I suddenly realized how inadequate I was as a counselor to this dying man. I offered him nothing, no comfort, no support, no empathy, no direction for him to face his death with understanding and dignity.

Death is the Edge of Mystery

Working for hospice was an entirely new venture for me. I thought I understood and possessed a talent for counseling people, addressing their concerns, and enabling them to resolve their issues. When I began to comprehend the mission of being a hospice chaplain, I found I lacked many skills. Most of my counseling experience was with folks with routine but resolvable concerns – marriage relationships, personal feelings of inadequacy, the need to feel accepted. The hospice patient was unique. Facing death is never routine. I realized that most of these patients were less concerned about nominal issues; rather, they confronted their eternal matters. Death is final and complete. There are no resolutions.

There is a difference, both in kind and in intensity, between caring giving and care receiving. Up to this time, I was a receiver of hospice care. While Ariel was going through the process of dying, the hospice people were extremely attentive and always present to her, as I will write later in this book. They were equally concerned and supportive of me twenty-four hours each day. I learned what it meant to be cared for - the constant support, the presence of people you can share your emotional state with, the feeling of knowing that whatever happens, you are not alone. As a chaplain, I was required to turn the other cheek, assume caregiving from a different perspective, and be a caregiver rather than a care receiver. I had to learn to offer the same kind of assistance, support, and empathic understanding to hospice patients that Ariel and I experienced from the hospice staff. It is a different experience. One does not assume you can give compassion just because you once received compassion.

Compassionate counseling was not entirely new to me; after all, I had spent the past thirty-two years in pastoral ministry. But hospice care is unique; it was different. No other psychosocial or medical program focuses principally on the terminally ill and their families, as does the hospice program. Their mandate is to offer palliative care, compassion, caring, and education strictly to the terminally ill. Hospice invests heavily in education that prepares the terminal patient and family for facing the inevitable, what to expect and how to deal with it. No other organization, do I know, devotes as much energy and expertise to this aspect of life as does hospice. It has become almost essential for the families of the dying. It demands the best of counseling.

I learned, painstakingly, but thoroughly the meaning of hospice spiritual care. It was intense, intentional, and comprehensive. Having been on the receiving end, I experienced spiritual care from the hospice staff. When I became a hospice chaplain, I had to re-learn spiritual care from a new perspective. Compassionate care takes on many roles.

Hospice care seeks to focus on the experience of dying and the spiritual implications of facing one's death. It begins with the assumption that the patient is facing imminent death and then seeks to make that experience as comfortable and meaningful as possible. It is into this circumstance that I now had to immerse myself. Those already doing hospice spiritual counseling willingly served as my mentors.

So, what is spiritual care all about?

What is spiritual care? Hospice counseling originates from a clear and concise understanding of spiritual care. The chaplain focuses on a distinct set of conditions. Perhaps these can best be described as follows: Spirituality gives meaning to a person's life. It has to do with how we live with and without a sense of hope, the content of our relationships, what we value, and the feeling of dignity.

- Spirituality addresses the things that are deeply felt and important to a person's life.

- A person's spirituality is the understanding of what brings meaning and purpose to life.

- Spirituality is different from religion; it probes the significance of life whereas religion is a set of practices specific to the person's faith.

- Spiritual care focuses on the person, not the disease.

The truth is that the day we receive a terminal prognosis is the day we enter completely unknown territory. The task placed before us is the challenge of finding the courage to face death's mystery. If there is to be meaning in life, we must somehow find meaning in death. I have always maintained that the Christian faith's central focus when it suggests an afterlife does so because it recognizes that no one is free to live fully now until they no longer fear death. ; The person has to accept death fully as a part of living.

When we tell people they are going to die, part of their work is to accept that. Learning to accept dying gives the patient a prolonged time to think about what they have done in life. A lot of times, patients begin to think, "I must have done something wrong. God must be punishing me. Why is it taking so long to die? What have I done? There must be something wrong with my faith because now I am scared to die." When people have died, we close the doors to prevent people from seeing the mortuary workers coming in to remove the body. The patients realize why those doors get shut. One woman told me, 'If I leave and go home, maybe I will not die."

Hope hospice chaplains provide support and an objective, a listening presence as the dying person and family consider questions about the purpose of life, suffering, need for forgiveness, and the progressive losses that accompany a severe illness. Contemplating one's life can help establish a person's legacy, how one lives on in the future, or how one wants to be remembered. Chaplains may also provide an honoring and caring presence for those unable to express their thoughts and feelings verbally.

At the time of Ariel's terminal sickness, I have to confess that I was not always conscious of spiritual issues that were either a part of her life or of my own. I unintentionally chose to suppress any spirituality that might have existed. When dealing with the terminal illness that Ariel was suffering, my most intense feelings focused on "how to resolve the problem." Facing potential death for me was like meeting a disease for which all efforts should go toward finding a cure. The feelings that surround the experience become intense. There is no time for reflection on such concerns as spiritual issues. There was lots of misplaced worry and anxiety, there was outright fear of losing a person, and a huge effort was extended to keep her comfortable. Pain frightened me, especially Ariel's. I had left over and little time and even less energy remaining to consider the spiritual side; to think about what brings meaning and purpose to Ariel's life. I assumed the role of "fixer;" nothing would deter my efforts to eliminate her pain and restore her health.

The difference between being a recipient of hospice care and providing hospice care came as a revelation to me. When I dealt with the terminal sickness that Ariel suffered, I felt I suffered right alongside her. I confess that I was not strong or confident throughout the ordeal. There were times I thought I never wanted this to happen. It was a dream, and eventually, I would wake up. At other times, I felt like a martyr, the person divinely chosen to provide total care for my wife despite what difficulty it might cause me. Living through her dying experience was a personal challenge; it was as if I was being punished because I had to care for her. I remember times vividly I felt cheated, that her sickness was depriving me of my future. Resentment began to rear its ugly head. I hated myself for suggesting this feeling, but it reared its head despite my protestations.

After Ariel passed and I became a hospice chaplain, the spiritual perspective was everything. The spiritual perspective was foremost in the dying experience. Once you are personally removed from the circumstance, it makes a difference, and you can look upon the situation from a professional objective viewpoint. As a chaplain, I intentionally attempted to ferret out from the patient issues relative to spiritual living. I would ask specifically, "What is most important to you right now?" or "where do you get your strength"? One question that always elicits a response, sometimes positive and other times negative is "How do you want to be remembered after you are gone?

Spirituality is defined differently by different people, but particular characteristic remains the same. I like the definition proposed by Daniel B. Hinshaw, in his article entitled "The Spiritual Needs of the Dying Patient. "Spirituality….is that which allows a person to experience transcendent meaning in life. This is often expressed as a relationship with God, but it can also be about nature, art, music, family or community – whatever beliefs and values give a person a sense of meaning and purpose in life." He further states that it is the lack of this sense of meaning in the face of terminal illness that creates the patient's spiritual distress. Hence, the hospice chaplain's task is to aid in the restoration and maintenance of the integrity of the spiritual life of the dying patient.

My task is manifold. Among the activities, I have assumed as a spiritual counselor is what we call "life review." Life review enables the patient to identify and reflect on what he/she has accomplished and created and what will be left behind as a legacy of that person's life. A second motivation is to enable the patient to rectify resentments. One of the priorities I discovered among terminally ill patients is the fear of not forgiving or not being forgiven of past offenses. Reconciliation is central to the work of the dying person. Reconciliation may or may not be associated with the person's religious beliefs; it stands by itself as a cleansing mechanism in preparation for the finality of death.

Spiritual care is not reserved solely for the dying; it must extend to the family and friends, the caretakers of the terminally ill. In my ministry, I found that at least half the time, resources, and efforts are directed to the family's spiritual crisis. Significant spiritual matters include but are not limited to the caretaker's ability to accept what is happening to the loved one, the ability to let go when the person has died, and the ability to experience empathy. Sometimes, I recognized that the caregiver's attitude changed during the disease. It might have begun in great anticipation of how fully the caretaker will take care of the patient. It often quickly dissolves into anger or resentment that the patient requires too much time and energy from the caretaker. Empathy on the part of the caretaker wanes and sometimes becomes completely lost or absent altogether. The chaplain must address this situation holistically for the welfare of both the patient and the caregiver.

Chapter 4

Does Caregiving Ever End

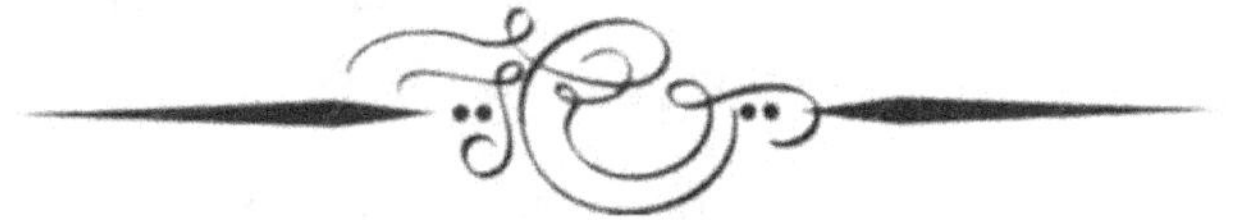

"There are only four kinds of people in the world. Those who have been caregivers. Those who are currently caregivers. Those who will be caregivers, and those who will need a caregiver."

- Rosalyn Carter

When I became a chaplain for Hospice, I realized that specific issues are more critical than other patients' issues. Among the most frequent questions asked, especially from patients' families, was, "Will caregiving ever end?"

Caregiving is not for sissies. There is work, and then there is hard work, then there is caregiving. Caregiving for the dying patient is incredibly stressful. It quickly takes its toll upon those souls' brave enough to undertake it.

I have worked all my life. Since the age of fourteen, I have worked hard each summer. Did things like selling vegetables at a roadside farm stand, was a lifeguard at a country club pool, drove a taxi on the beach, and once, but only briefly, I hung rugs to dry in a commercial laundry. I thought this was all hard work, but what did I know then. I was untested and young.

After graduate school, I served as a minister for thirty years in a variety of churches. I worked hard at this vocation. My kids never understood that being a minster was work

"You just go to meetings," dad, "they remarked when asked what I did for a living. "And then you talk for twenty minutes once a week on Sunday mornings."

Later in life, when I had the opportunity to become a hospice chaplain after Ariel died, my perspective on work changed drastically. I met people (mostly family members) who were assigned, sometimes by default or sometimes by intention, to be the caregivers for their loved ones who were hospice patients. When they took on the task, they pleaded ignorance of the responsivities required and were astonished at the amount of work necessary.

Family caregivers providing palliative care necessitate unrelenting vigilance. They are required to provide continual adaptation to the challenging dependency needs of their ill and dying family members. How people respond to this overwhelming task can be overwhelming. – burnout, guilt, physical and mental exhaustion, stress, anxiety, and depression are just a few of the detriments that contribute toward making caregiving among the most difficult of human endeavors.

I soon learned of the manifold tasks of those who care for the dying. The caregiver is required to provide several forms of care to the loved-one during the dying process. More than any other type of caregiving, the caretaker of the dying must work tirelessly to provide comprehensive care that treats the whole patient, including mental, emotional, physical, spiritual, and social care. By caring for the whole patient, the caregiver seeks to provide the best quality of life possible under the circumstances. The caregiver's goal is to make the patient comfortable, calm, and at peace, easing the transition to death. While the loved-one may feel at ease, the caregiver may be experiencing fatigue, stress, and anxiety. The strenuous role of the caregiver leaves little room for self-care during the dying process.

Most caregivers either don't get the support they need or try to do more than they can. A variety of side effects result from exhausted caregivers – lack of sleep, social withdrawal, feelings of wanting to hurt themselves or the person for whom they are caring, irritability, and alcohol or drug abuse.

Don't expect appreciation for your caregiving. Dying people are sometimes crabby or even cruel, since they may be responding in fear of the dying process or the physical pain of dying. They often react in anger and argumentation. They want to blame you, the caregiver. Don't take the bait. Even when you feel frustrated by the dying person's actions or behaviors, avoid getting into arguments that you will regret someday. There is a constant feeling of guilt. Caregivers presume that all their time must be spent on caring for the patient, but they are constantly plagued by feelings of inadequacy, or feeling they are not suitable to the task; not living up to their expectations of being a satisfactory caregiver; a dilemma that is impossible to remedy.

From the above caregiving description, I hope you begin to understand that caregiving is "work" of the most problematic that any person might have to undertake. It will fully challenge you and will test your patience and stamina to the nth degree. Survival will not be easy. Only those with durable mental and physical qualities dare apply.

Now that I have your attention let me explain. As the chaplain for a hospice, as much of my time was spent in consultation with family members (particularly spouses) as was spent with the patient. Despite the altruistic motivation, there comes a time when all caregivers wonder, "Will this ever end?"

Before contacting hospice, most caregivers would have been devastated by the thought of a loved one dying. Their motivation would have been one of pure altruism; that no matter the circumstance, they would happily assume the role of caretaker, never balking from responsibility, nary a thought about abandoning the task. Perish the thought that Mom might need nursing home assistance. I have heard the adamant statements many times; "I aint going to put Mom in one of those nursing homes." The caregiver decides, usually out of guilt, to take care of the patient him/herself and keeps on keeping on.

Soon, however, reality creeps in. Life as they knew it changes radically. Exhaustion sets in, resentment rears its ugly head, and questions of adequacy abound. "Why do I have to do this every day? Maybe it would be better to send Mom to a nursing home? Dad demands so much of my time." The caregivers' relationship with family and friends takes on a new dimension. It begins to deteriorate. The caregiver yearns for the past, begins to resent the present, and looks to the future with skepticism. "Is there no end?" There is no way of knowing how long the role of caregiver will last.

When the hospice patient has declined significantly that they no longer resemble the person they used to be, it can be heartbreaking to imagine prolonging such a life. Patients can become demanding, abusive, demented, and even violent. These circumstances can take a heavy emotional toll on the patient and the caregiver. The medical community has done everything possible but has run out of options, so the caregiver starts thinking how nice it would be if the hospice patient just went to sleep one night and never woke up. After all, they are going to die anyway. This way, the caregiver gets back his/ her life.

"I really wish mom would pass, sooner rather than later" was the expressed feeling of one of my patients. "Don't get me wrong, all the doctors who helped care for my mother were kind and compassionate and truly concerned for her well-being. But their first concern was always dealing with the physical concerns that would prolong her life. The doctor's task is to worry about prolonging life, not worry about the quality of life. That was the hard part for me."

When these thoughts creep into the caregiver's mind, the immediate reaction is often extreme guilt and shame. Openly the caregiver could never admit to these feelings. Underneath, however, they are real feelings that fester and grow. What is essential to understand is that they are just feelings; it doesn't mean the caregiver will act on them. To say this job is difficult is an understatement. We begin to think about when the responsibilities will end, but mostly, it remains just a thought.

Because caregivers occasionally have thoughts of wishing the loved one would die does not mean they are horrible, cruel people. They are not thinking about "hurrying up the process." This wish is more of a fantasy; they would just like to have their lives back the way they were before this all happened. They wish their loved one would experience healing and return to normal as well – mentally and physically healthy and independent, the way they used to be. Caregivers are humans, not saints.

Although most caregivers will not voice this sentiment for fear of how others will react to it, I believe most caregivers entertain the thought at some time. Having your life turn into something beyond what you felt you could handle can be distressing.

Most people are decent folks who care deeply about the plight of their parents, friends, spouse, or children who face a terminal disease. With few exceptions, people take on caring for a loved one with a terminal illness out of love and a strong sense of obligation. We convince ourselves that we are truly altruistic, and caregiving is a noble undertaking. Our help is needed so we jump in with both feet and the best of intentions. Good intentions are not always sufficient for the task.

However, we are completely oblivious to the full responsibility; that caretaking may last for months, perhaps even years, and will necessitate a great amount of time and energy. It doesn't occur to us that this commitment could jeopardize our traditional relationships, careers, health, and finances.

Many families are suddenly thrust into caregiving roles by default. The loved ones – spouse, child, the parent, or best friend – no longer can safely live by themselves, but nobody wants to take responsibility for putting that person in a "home." So, a family member steps up or is nominated to manage the care that is needed.

People are on an adrenaline high when making that decision - it seems appropriate, is best for the patient, and the person assigned as caregiver is deemed capable. The caregiver is eventually left alone as the rest of the family goes back to their previous lives. Caregiver isolation sets in quickly.

Reality sets in. The one person designated to manage the patient realizes the enormity of caring for the patient as well as living her own life – managing a career, a family, paying bills, meeting doctor's appointments, changing adult diapers, providing medications, and a whole host of other necessary tasks. Is it any wonder that resentments begin to rise? Real-life is not as the caregiver imagined it might be when taking on the responsibility of the caregiver.

After years as a hospice chaplain, I encountered this attitude of looming resentment among various patients and under differing circumstances. When that occurred, It reminded me of when I experienced the same attitude as I encountered my own experience of living with Ariel's death and dying.

Mrs. Howards Story

Mrs. Howard, the wife of a patient of mine was in the throes of dealing with her husband's severe dementia. According to her, he had become a "changed" person. Before the onset of this disease, he was a decorated Air Force veteran, a great-looking hombre, with lots of charm and charisma. They lived a storied life together ; tales of domestic and international travel, dinner parties, relaxing together at their waterfront home, children who were achievers, and grandchildren visit bringing delight to their lives. They lived life to the fullest as if each day was to be their last. One day it became their last.

Mr. Howard's dementia came on fast and aggressively. It appeared to her, his wife, that one day he was her normal husband, and the next day he was entirely in the throes of severe dementia. An immediate and radical change, hardly noticed until completed. He was a stranger in her house, unrecognizable.

She sought treatment. She refused to acknowledge that their lives were undergoing an irreversible and fundamental transformation. She found no potential treatment. She realized she confronted a physical and personality change that could not, would not, be reversed no matter how hard she prayed it would.

She was at her wit's end. She confided in me one day. "I feel so guilty, but sometimes I wish he would die sooner rather than later."

"What brings this on?" I asked.

"He is not himself. He is not the man I married, and I feel sure that if he had his wits about him, he would not want to live like this."

"It must be hard to know for sure what he must want for himself," I reminded her. "Maybe, just maybe, he would choose to be here with you." I shared with her some thoughts. "One thing we feel certain about with dementia patients is that they do not lose the ability to feel things – joy, anger, frustration. I know it must be difficult for you to know his needs since he can't tell you himself."

"I can tell when he is angry, even though he doesn't use his words," she said

"We can only guess," I responded. "When he refuses food, he is either not hungry or confused. When he is agitated, how do we know if it's not his pain? It's a crapshoot much of the time. We got to consider the possibility that he is aware of his surroundings and finds comfort and joy knowing you are present even though he can't tell you."

"But most times," she responded, "he doesn't even know who I am. He forgets my name. He doesn't respond to anything I suggest; he just stares at me like I am a stranger." She went to the kitchen and poured herself a cup of coffee. Her husband remained sleeping on the couch. "He hates it when I try to shower him. He fights me like a banshee, as if I am the enemy. I know he does not want to hurt me. He would never hurt me if he were in his right mind."

"With hospice, we can help keep him physically comfortable." I reminded her. "We can do that right up to the end. I guess what I am trying to say is that he is only half your problem; I understand that the other half is your mental state. It must be difficult for you to have to give up so much of your life; it's demanding and tiresome work to care for him, I understand. But recognize your feelings for what they are. It doesn't mean you are going to act on them, and they are just feelings that you have."

"Why does he resist me and at times even become openly angry with me? He scares me."

Mrs. Howard's queries about wishing her husband would pass on sooner rather than later persisted. Each visit, she shared more feelings but became more comfortable about having the feelings. Of course, she never gave any indication that she would act on these feelings and continued, to the best of my knowledge, to provide excellent care for her husband. In her estimate, she predicted he would hang on for a few more years. She committed herself to care for him for the duration. But she reiterated that she would not have to go that road alone and wanted assurance that hospice would stick by her.

Mrs. Howard is not unique. Over time I have come across many situations that reflect a similar circumstance. After an initial period of tolerance and flexibility, the spouse and/or children begin to resent the total focus on the patient. All involved feel shortchanged, and yet they continue to insist, "we can't put dad in a home." The primary caregiver acquiesces, partially out of feelings of guilt, and life keeps on keeping on.

As the demands on the caregiver continue to escalate and more and more time and energy are required, exhaustion sets in, and less energy is available for family and friends. Resentments begin to emerge about the present. The future is imagined with skepticism. This morbid, but the realistic realization, leads caregivers to wish for a conclusion to their situation.

When the loved ones are in pain, depressed, demanding, abusive, demented, and sometimes violent, it takes a heavy emotional toll. A great deal of effort is needed to keep them calm, provide for their comfort, or maintain their contentment. The medical community has done all it could, including the services of hospice, so even her friends begin thinking, "How nice if Mr. Howard just went to sleep one night and didn't wake up. He would be at peace, and Mrs. Howard would get her life back somewhat." When these thoughts creep into the caregiver's mind, the reaction is one of guilt and shame. But they are faced with a grueling challenge, like running a marathon when they get so exhausted all they can think of is getting to the finish line and ending the anguish. We begin to think about when our responsibilities will come to an end.

Caregivers who experience these feelings are not terrible people. They don't get consumed with thoughts about speeding up the process. Few people ever get to the point of articulating these feelings; they remain in the back of their minds. To express them openly is to risk that others will think of them as cold-hearted and callous. Most of these caregivers are feeling overwhelmed and seemingly out of options. They just don't know what to do.

Mrs. Howard is comforted by knowing that she is not crazy, she is not merciless, and she is not callous just because of the normal feelings she is experiencing.

Mrs. Farnsworth Story

Mrs. Farnsworth was the caretaker of her mother. "Yes, I wanted to care for Mom," she told me when I asked what led to her ailing mother being at her home. Mom was a dementia patient in addition to another comorbidity; a supplementary disease that qualifies for hospice in addition to her primary diagnosis. "I volunteered. I knew I could do it. I think I have a better temperament than my siblings."

"How has this worked out for you?" I asked, knowing that caretaking can be a demeaning and demanding task. I try to gauge a sense of how caretakers perceive the job by asking, "Are you doing alright?"

After thirty years of hospice care, the folks at Hope Hospice recognized that caretaking, although extremely important, can also be extremely demanding. It often ends in resentments of all kinds, sometimes even resenting the patients who require caretaking because of their burdens on the caretaker. Caregiving sapps energy and exhausts enthusiasm. Guilt sets in for the caretaker. Despite begrudging the problematic work of caretaking, remnants of blame linger. The caretaker is never content that his/her efforts are sufficient.

Hospice address this issue of caregiver fatigue through a variety of responsive programs; the most utilized is respite care. If and when the primary caretaker feels overwhelmed and begins to lose the ability or willingness to care for the patient, hospice, in tangent with the caretaker, has the option of placing the patient in a cooperating nursing facility for five consecutive days each month. The patients' family along with hospice staff, mutually decide eligibility. Hospice provides transportation to and from the facility. One or more of our staff visits daily. This program is often a God-sent to families struggling with the demands of caretaking. Upon first hearing the suggestion of respite care, most families refuse. Feelings of guilt for abandoning their loved ones seem overwhelming and unnatural, but eventually, after consideration, most chose the respite care option.

I previously described this program to Mrs. Farnsworth. Her reaction was typical.

"I could never do that," she exclaimed in no uncertain terms.

"Why would that be so difficult?" I asked her.

"I would feel so guilty. I could never stand myself." She made it sound almost immoral. She continued to state more explanations of self-loathing and personal affronts for even considering the option of respite.

"That would make me feel like I was abandoning Mom. How could anyone do that?"

I acknowledged her feeling but added, "It would only be for a short time, and then you bring her home again. You assure her that she will come home after the five days." I added that if she planned to continue care for her mother, it might be wise to take care of herself. An exhausted caregiver is of little value.

She acknowledged my thoughts but still reneged. "I get tired, but I still want to do this, "she concluded. After a short pause, she added, "Can I tell you something else?"

"Absolutely."

"My brothers and sister come by once in a while to visit with Mom. They don't live too far from me. What bothers me is that after asking me to be the one to care for mom, they start to get critical. When they visit, they say things like 'Mom doesn't eat enough' or 'she looks like she is losing weight' or 'she looks ragged.' The other day when my brother was here, he had the gall to ask me if I was treating her well." She paused for a moment and took a sip from the cup she had been holding. "There seems to be always something they think I should be doing differently, but they never volunteer to take care of her even for a short time. It's always me. They are never satisfied with what I do. They still want her to stay here. That bothers me," she said as she finished her explanation.

She was clearly expressing her annoyance. She began to shed tears. She reached for the Kleenex from a nearby table. "Excuse me," she said. "I don't mean to upset you."

"No, you're fine," I responded. I asked the obvious question. "It sounds like siblinmgs are not willing to take any responsibly but are more willing to criticize you. I think I hear you saying that makes you resentful."

"Yes, but I know I shouldn't feel that way." More tears began to flow and again, she reached for the Kleenex.

"How you feel is just how you feel (I am good at profound thoughts). You don't need to make judgments about your feelings," I wanted to provide Mrs. Farnsworth with some comforting and reassuring words at this point. I felt a situation like this called for comforting hugs, but professionals have to act with restraint.

She dried her tears. I asked her, "Do you feel good about your caring? Do you think you are doing a good job?"

"Yes, I think I do a good job. Mom is doing as well as can be expected. But the criticism from them begins to wear on me. I feel resentful but don't want to feel like that."

Suddenly I felt a great urge to plunge in and offer some counsel. I like to think I am offering help remedying her circumstance but can't help feeling that my analysis may just be me talking to hear myself talk. Nevertheless, I offered the following:

"You are in charge. They asked you to take care of Mom. You can't have a committee to do that sort of thing. One person needs to be in charge. Others can help along the way, but you should not allow them to be critical of something they refuse responsibility. If you are right, you take the credit. If you are wrong, you take the blame. And don't be afraid to tell them so. Let them know you appreciate their suggestions but that you and you alone will decide Mom's care. Or let somebody else take over. Have mom move in with them. Until that day, make sure they know you are boss."

It felt good to get that off my chest. I took a great leap of faith with that admonishment, for better or worse. I did realize that if she took my advice and it backfired or caused even more divisiveness among the family members, it would be my fault; I needed to take responsibility for failure. I was willing to do that .

Caregiver stress- A Few Essentials

Part of the stress comes from the uncertainty of a situation. The caregiver may understand that if this is a terminal illness, death is near, but it is usually impossible to know when. The caregiver may worry each day about the outcome and what medical emergency they may need to cope with today.

Caregivers may also face financial problems and stress. Many have given up their full-time jobs to care for their family member. There may be mounting medical bills to pay for. On top of providing day-to-day medical and living care, the caregiver may need to cope with daily phone calls from bill collectors or budgeting limited amounts of money to try to cover expenses.

Caregivers may need to help other family members cope with the situation or play referee with feuding relatives. Family disagreements on medical care or other decisions can create friction, adding to the stress caregivers may feel.

Caregivers often put off taking care of themselves. They may feel (or be) on call 24 hours a day, or they may never have a break from their duties. Caregivers often have interrupted sleep, little time to relax, and less time to pursue their interests or spend time with their friends.

On top of all of this, caregivers must deal with their own emotions of facing death daily as well as mourning the upcoming loss of their loved one. Some studies show the rate of depression in caregivers of terminally ill patients to be as high as fifty percent.

Caregivers may need to make decisions that make him or her uncomfortable or were decisions once made by the patient. Not only must the decisions be made, but the caregiver must deal with the inability of the patient, maybe the result of Alzheimer's disease. (Caregivers of patients with Alzheimer's have more symptoms of stress and depression than those caring for patients with other physical illnesses.)

Suggestions for Support

For those in a situation where they identify they have feelings of resentment toward the person they are caring for, they can seek some reprieve by attending to various aspects of the circumstances - the depression, the lack of understanding, and the absence of support. I suggest the following, not as exhaustive ways for a reprieve, but suggested means for coping.

Stress: Unchecked stress often contributes to caregiver burnout. Get a checkup from your doctor and don't forget to mention to him/her the details of your circumstance. Medications, if necessary, can be of great assistance.

Respite Care: Take time off and go somewhere; disconnect from caregiving for a short period. Utilize the respite care option of hospice.

Find a sanctuary: Be alone, even if for a short period. Go to the library, local coffee house, swimming pool, bike ride, long walk or ask a friend to take over for thirty minutes or longer, whatever time they will afford you..

Support Group: I can't stress strongly enough the value of sharing with others in similar circumstances. There is a world of knowledge out there that is part of others' repertoire living with the same circumstance. Comradery makes a big difference.

Chapter 5

Ariel's Story – Leaning to the Left

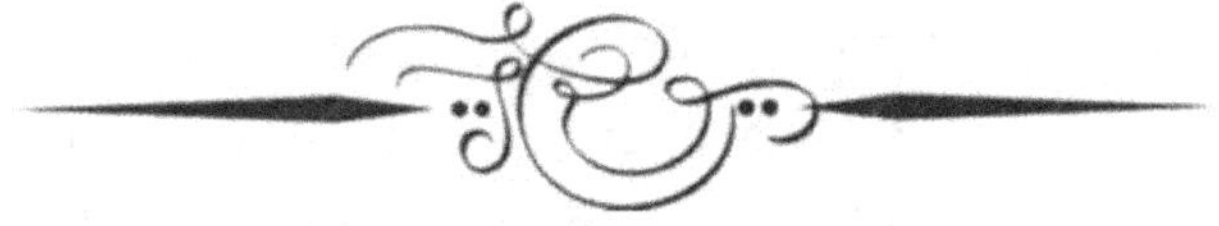

"A woman is like a tea bag- You can't tell how strong she is until you put her in hot water."

- Eleanor Roosevelt

The first weeks after returning from our Disney World venture with the grandchildren, Ariel occasionally mentioned that her back still hurt.

"Nothing drastic," she remarked. "Probably from carrying Sophia around Disney World."

"Well, you did carry the kid a lot," I responded. "She's not that heavy, and she seemed to like that you held her.." There were other times when Ariel commented on her back pain, never a complaint, just a matter-of-fact explanation. I paid little attention as I thought "back pain" from carrying a kid. How bad can it be? It will pass.

Every Fourth of July, our entire family plus a few friends gathered at a camp just outside our town. The camp is located on a river and has a family-friendly pool. Regular student camp sessions disband over the Fourth of July weekend. It's an excellent opportunity for a family reunion free from the hassles of overcrowded public places during the holiday. We gather together and plan our celebration at the empty camp.

Ariel had always been possessive of organizing food purchases and food preparations for these types of family experiences. It's her way of showing love – food. Menus were planned with great pride keeping in mind the diverse needs of those present - kids, teenagers, adults, grandparents. Ariel assigned our adult kids different parts of the food purchases and preparations, always under her supervision, however.

This Fourth of July was different. "Since my back is hurting," she said, "I think I will ask the kids to make most of the menu preparations and food purchase." Her request came as a complete surprise, an enormous concession on her part and a serious departure from the norm.

"You are going to let the kids do all the work for the food," I asked. "How come?"

She reiterated that her back was bothering her, and she just didn't feel like doing it all herself. For me, that was a clue that something was wrong.

It was a gloriously sunny and warm weekend, perfect for hanging out together, beer-drinking while sitting in the river to keep cool, hiking the paths in the woods, and lounging by the pool with the younger children. I noticed that Ariel did not want to come to the pool. I remembered that she loved to sit in the shallow end of the pool with her youngest grandchild and splash around while the two giggled together. She wanted to stay at the cabin.

"It's my back," she said. "It's bothering me."

I started remembering how many times she commented on her backaches over the past few weeks, And I gave it little attention. Not now

"This has been going on too long to ignore," I said to her. "When we get home, can we make an appointment with the doctor, please?"

"I suppose so," she responded. Ariel never liked when I suggested that she take care of herself. I thought it a trait unique to nurses. Caring for others was expected, but for one's self, caring was not characteristic of nurses.

Tuesday evening at dinner, Ariel told me she had made an appointment with the doctor. After a brief conversation with this doctor, she said he referred her to a specialist who he thought could do better in diagnosing her problem,

"When is the appointment," I asked her? "Who is it with?"

"Day after tomorrow – Thursday. I can't remember his name, but he is in San Antonio."

"Can I go with you?"

"Sure"

There was silence for a while as we consumed our meal. I could sense Ariel was worried, but would not admit it. She has a sixth sense when she feels something is not as it should be but says nothing about it. Nonetheless, I suspected she was concerned.

"Do you think there is something wrong, or is it just from carrying Sophia," I asked her

"If that were the case, I should feel better by now. It's been a few weeks."

On Thursday afternoon, we both showed up at the specialist's office. He seemed competent and pleasant. I reserved judgment and trusted our internist's ability to make proficient referrals.

"We should take some x-rays," he suggested. He then proceeded to ask Ariel some questions. He examined her back by probing with his fingers attempting to identify the exact location of her pain. "We can take the x-rays right now, and I can read them while you are here." He suggested. Ariel agreed.

Ariel disappeared into a back room and, fifteen minutes later, reappeared in the waiting room. Then the doctor called us into the examination room. Ariel sat down, and I remained standing. The x-rays were up on a lighted board where we could see them.

"Can't see anything significant," he stated while he looked closely at the x-rays. He pointed to some areas on Ariel's back, indicating there was nothing remarkable to see. "It's probably a strain. You said you carried your grandchild; perhaps that is what caused the strain. That may be the cause. It's a lot like tennis elbow," he said. "You have to suffer through it for a while, and it should go away."

For the first time in the last few days, I saw Ariel's face relax. "That sounds like good news," I told her.

"Yes, I think I worried because I have never had back problems before, so why now? I feel a bit relieved."

Her back pain hung on for the next few weeks. She continued to work for Hope Hospice as usual, never complained, but did notice that although it didn't diminish in intensity, neither did it increase. It was a subject we both tried to ignore, thinking the doctor must be right. If we don't talk about it, it will go away eventually.

Ariel's assignment as a hospice nurse required her to lift patients and move them to a wheelchair or assist them in getting to the bathroom or simply changing from the bed to a chair. She understood the mechanics of proper lifting, but still, it took considerable energy and muscle strain. When she did mention her back as still hurting, it was always a matter of factual information and never as a complaint. Complaining had no place in Ariel's character.

Although I was aware of her constant back pain, I still thought it was temporary. It didn't need any special attention. It would moderate, eventually, fade away all on its own given time. That was my expectation, and my expectations began to take precedent over the truth. For the first time, feelings of resentment crept in. I was starting to feel like she was an intrusion in my life; her ailments kept us from going and doing what we had planned. Resentment reared its ugly head. I saw it coming but couldn't stop it. Internally, my emotions felt like a roller-coaster, sometimes empathetic and other times selfish. My thoughts turned to time; how much time will it take before we (I meant me) can get on with life as usual?

Ariel had similar thoughts. She tried to focus minimally on her back pain, paid slight attention, and continued to function as if there was no need for concern. She worked every day despite that her back continued to ache. Still no complaining, no feeling sorry for herself. Ariel just would never be like that.

My first realization that Ariel's back pain was more than just a simple back spasm or common lower back sprain occurred when I noticed that she started taking ibuprofen pills on a regular schedule, three or four times each day. Taking pills was unusual. I had not known her to be a pill taker unless under dire circumstances. She avoided medications like the plague. The only exceptions were calcium pills, and a medication called Fosamax to help with female aging osteoporosis. Both were to slow down bone loss after menopause. She had taken them for a few years, but nothing else.

I confronted her one night with this concern. "You are taking a considerable amount of ibuprofen lately," I told her. "Is it because of your back pain?"

"Not a lot," she insisted. My comment probably felt critical to her or as a judgment indicated by the tone by which she answered. She continued with an explanation. "It's because my back just doesn't seem to get any better, and it bothers me a lot. I need the meds to get through the workday," she told me. "I'm still hoping it's just a sprain like the doctor said, but some days I wonder. But stop worrying." It was most important to her that I not worry.

"Do you think we should go to a different doctor; get a second opinion," I asked her? "How long do you want to wait? How long can you live with the pain?" I think I was also asking myself – how long will I have to deal with your problem?

"I want to wait a little longer." Ariel had a strong personality. She could not be tempted differently very easily. Her stubborn streak was difficult to overcome. She was not to be persuaded.

I started to take more notice of her behavior since I observed the increased medications. She walked with a slight but discerning lean in her gait. Her lean was slightly to the left. She was not standing straight. She swung her left arm across her midsection as if reaching to relieve an annoyance in her side.

"You look like you are walking crooked," I said to her one evening while she was smoking in the garage. "Can you stand up straight?" She tried, but she continued to lean to the left as if bent sideways at the hip.

"I guess I am," she acknowledged. "When I try to straighten up, it hurts my back even more," She tried to stand straight, but grimaced, stopped, and relaxed.

"You're leaning to the left again, "I observed, No response, only another unsuccessful attempt to right herself.

Chapter 6

Angry with God

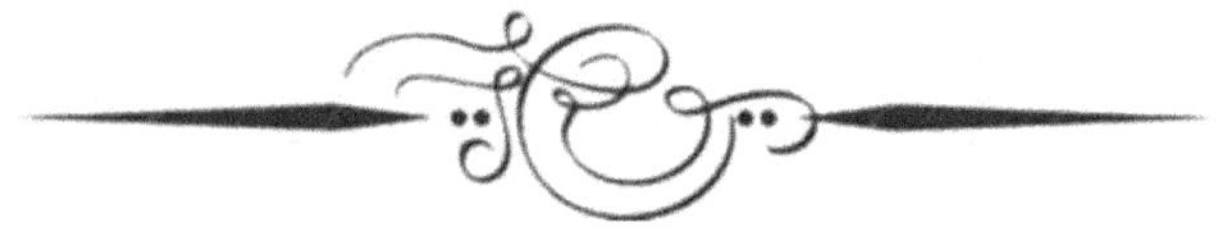

"In my frustration, I turned my sights on God and hydroplaned through all kinds of prayers: name-it-and claim-it declarations, lamentations, pleas for mercy, bargaining, and even trying to put Him on guilt trips. None of it worked. Things only got worse-especially the side effects of the medications – and what hurt the most was that God could heal it instantly, but for some reason, He was choosing not to"

- Anonymous Patient Response

Resentments felt by hospice patients include those of the caregiver but also grievances of the patient. The question arises, "Why Me?" Only God has that answer. When all else fails, we tend to blame God.

Anger with God is as old as time. Hardly ever did I have a patient who did not express anger at God for his/her circumstance. Patients expressing anger when facing death are not unique. Anger at God, blaming God when things go wrong is symptomatic of all society, even those who do not believe in God. People get mad at God all the time for many reasons, even about ordinary, daily disappointments. General psychology reveals that being angry at God is a collective human emotion that stems from the belief that God is responsible for both good and bad experiences.

Many of my patients became angry with God because they saw God as personally responsible for adverse events in life. They interpreted His intentions as cruel, thinking God had abandoned them, betrayed them, or mistreated them. Not surprisingly, the intensity of their pain is matched by the intensity of their anger toward God. We wonder why we "deserve" such a personal tragedy. "Why me, God?"

But no one "deserves" tragedy. That is why we are angry with God. Most of us grew up with the notion inherited from our parents and religious teachers that if we were "good," God would preserve us from bad things. Bad things only happened to the "wicked." This well-meant teaching turns out to be false! As we grow up, we discover painfully that bad things happen to all people, whether people are judged as "good" or "wicked."

When confronted by this attitude from a hospice patient (and sometimes by a family member), I had to struggle to respond appropriately. It was never sufficient to point to scripture which tells us,

"But now you also, put them all aside: anger, wrath, malice, slander, and abusive speech from your mouth."

(Colossians 3:8).

But if you're honest, your reaction to this verse is probably, "I agree! But, really, *how* do you do it?" It's easy to say, "Put all your anger and abusive speech aside." But it's another thing when the anger is overwhelming.

When someone's struggling with anger at God, rather than referring him to scripture texts, make sure you first have his ear. Take a walk with him as a friend. Acknowledge the value of his being honest about his struggle with God. Affirm his current conviction that life in a fallen world can be difficult and deeply disappointing. Beyond these general guidelines, it's hard to know how you might script that first relational step where you're trying to build some trust with a patient. Yet, your purpose is clear: you're trying to be the friend who cares about a person who feels like nobody cares about him.

Mr. Williams' Story

The morning hospice report indicated that I was assigned a new patient overnight. He was in the intensive care unit of the local hospital. Many times, we admit to the hospital because of a complication with their disease. However, while in the hospital, they are advised that the disease has progressed beyond recovery and are given a new diagnosis of being terminal. The attending physician will recommend that the family admit them to hospice.

Hearing the word "hospice" can be a traumatic time for both patient and family; They construe it as a death decree. Who wants to hear that death is forthcoming? In addition to the diagnosis, they are usually informed that the hospital can no longer treat them. As soon as possible, the hospital dismisses them. This means they go to a nursing facility or their own home where hospice becomes the caretaker. There is indignity attached to being kicked out of a hospital.

When told of a terminal disease diagnosis, not all patients are anxious. Some receive the news stoically; they appear unimpressed by such a critical proclamation, an assertion that generally elicits grave concern. "So, I got a death sentence. We all have to die sometime," is a reaction I have gotten from more than one of my patients.

Some feign flat-out denial, although it's sometimes difficult to distinguish between stoicism and denial. For those who receive the news of their illness as an abrupt death warrant, their reaction is two parts despondency, one-part gloom, and a sprinkle of anguish thrown in for flavor. "Oh my God, why me? How can this be? I don't believe this." My task as a chaplain is to ferret out their emotions and offer counsel toward understanding and coping with strong personal feelings. The gravity of these feelings significantly affects their spiritual lives.

This morning my patient was Mr. Williams, a middle-aged married man with children. Mr. Williama was quick to disclose his feelings about living the American dream; living a life that reflects attaining most all of his goals and ambitions; that is until he gets his terminal diagnosis. Upon meeting him for the first time, it was clear that he was in denial, refusing to either believe or accept the inevitable. Only six months remained to his life expectancy.

"Tell me this isn't happening" were his first words when I introduced myself as a hospice chaplain. I neither confirmed nor denied his proclamation. "This is not what I had hoped for," he continued. "I'm not sure what to believe, the doctor or my intuition."

"What's your intuition?" I asked.

"I am not done living. Certainly not ready to die. I can't believe that they can't cure this disease since I have been so healthy all my life. I mean, what about all this miracle medicine I keep hearing about; is it all bullshit?" I could only listen since I had no answer. I wanted to offer him comfort

The hospital sent Mr. Williams home. Hospitals are disposed to discharge patients who are dying. Medical science deals with curing disease, not with the dying. They offer little assistance as it is not part of the Hippocratic Oath to allow someone to die in their presence.

My next visit occurred at his home. Mr. Williams confessed that he only reluctantly "allowed" hospice to be his partner in this journey. "I am not sure I need hospice," were the first words out of his mouth upon my arrival. His language and demeanor implied that his disease might stay behind at the hospital if he got home. Denial remained a strong motivator for him.

We got to talking with each other. I was impressed by his robust evangelical Christian beliefs. He was unwavering in the adamancy of his faith, a trait that would come back to haunt him. Yet, he admitted to presently undergoing some serious faith apprehension and confusion.

When the awareness of his terminal disease diagnosis sunk in, he became extremely distraught and agitated. He told me how he reacted to an overwhelming impulse to go to his church, "probably," he said, "because the possibility of his death frightened him," and he was angry. He shared with me what happened.

He entered the sanctuary and stood directly in front of the altar.

"You can't do this to me," he said. "It's just not fair." Those were his first words but not his last. "You're a fraud," he continued, "a phony God. Every time someone finds contentment and peace in life, a little bit of happiness, you take it all away. I am so angry with you."

"I felt completely fatigued," he later told me. The disease had depleted his strength, and his outburst of anger toward God exhausted his forte. He said he then dropped to his knees, buried his head in his hands, and sobbed uncontrollably.

I realized it was a spiritual heart attack, indeed. Metaphorically the heart is the seat of our emotions. Heart disease can be spiritual as well as physical. To suffer from a hardened heart, the consequence of emotional resentment or regret causes as much pain and grief as the worst case of occluded arteries. Sometimes it festers for decades undetected. Resentment and regret can erupt suddenly and without warning. Like a weed, its roots spread deep into our spirit, infecting the soul like a plant with poisonous fruit. Worst of all, resentment focuses on the people we know and love the most.

I got to thinking about resentment, particularly after Mr. Williams confessed that he resented his son. They were estranged for many years, initially because of unresolved slights on each other's value system. Resentments often emerge with terminal patients. The "disease progression" seems to allow time for reflection. Mr. Williams was one of those fraught with bitterness, an experience that decimated his life as he struggled with his relationship with his son.

I continued my conversation with him as he talked about his son.

"I want him to know that I love him," he told me, "but I am afraid if I make contact now after so long, he might think I just want to interfere in his life again."

I was puzzled. "Why on earth would you feel that way?" I asked.

"Because that is what split us apart in the first place. He accused me of interfering too much in his life. We have different values, and we seldom, if ever agree." He paused. He seemed to be contemplating some thought before he continued. "I find myself imposing my opinions on what he should be doing or not doing and then criticizing whatever he chooses. He thinks I never approve of anything in his life, and he is probably right. I always interfered because I thought I knew what was best for him. (A reflection of his unwavering faith affirmations). We would always end up arguing"

"Arguing is talking," I reminded him. "It keeps the contact open."

"But that's not the way I want it to be. It's too late now."

"Never too late," I affirmed.

"I'm getting too tired to deal with this stuff," was his considered response.

We broke off the conversation, and shortly afterward, I decided to leave. I felt we made no progress. Our conversation just reiterated old bias and misunderstandings as well as misplaced anger. We did not break new ground. I was anxious to visit again soon and told him so.

I asked him. "Can I come back next Tuesday?"

"Yeah," he replied. "But you might be wasting your time."

Reflecting on our first visit, I ruminated on what I remembered from past conversations with patients who expressed similar feelings. The stronger the love, I remembered thinking, the greater the potential for resentment. Because we love God so much, as Mr. Williams did, we are then prone to resent God equally as much. Without a substantial commitment of love, there seems to be little incentive to feel resentment. Perhaps that is why the little girl who was angry with her father because he did not allow her to watch her favorite television program wrote him a note that said, "Dear Daddy. I hate you. Love, Rebecca."

Often the indignity of being hurt is misdirected. We are not sure with whom we are angry or who to blame for our painful circumstance, so we take it out on God. We claim to love God but love and hate are not opposites; they are different sides of the same coin. The opposite of hate is indifference. Hate is too powerful an emotion to carry with us for a long time. It exhausts us completely as it did with Mr. Williams. Eventually, our strong feelings of animosity dissolve into indifference. We don't care.

At our next visit together, despite his protestations, I suggested he didn't care anymore. He denied that assumption. He spoke adamantly

"You are always asking me what is most important to me right now," he said. "I can stand whatever physical pain might be coming my way. I don't want to die. I still think it is unfair." He paused for a few moments and then continued. "I am afraid of regrets. I have a terrible fear of dealing with them like the ones about which we have talked. I need to get rid of these before I die. I think about them all the time. When I think about regrets and about dying at the same time, it feels overwhelming. I know I don't have much time left to live, and I don't want to die feeling resentful." Tears formed in his eyes, and his speech was tentative.

"I understand what you are saying," I responded. "What do you want to do about this?"

He did not answer right away. I suspected what he wanted- reconciliation with his son, but realized it had to be his idea. To be powerfully therapeutic for him, he had to take the personal initiative to overcome his resentments. Otherwise, he was not responsible for anything I might suggest. Again, I said, what do you want to do?"

Resentment, I think, is a substantial barrier to positive spiritual formation. Resentment may begin focusing on a particular person but soon becomes generalized. We become angry persons. Anger dominates our personality. The bitterness becomes internalized, a kind of addiction we can't shake. As with any addiction, resentment consumes our life. We live to vent our anger. According to a friend of mine, "Resentments are when we rent space in our heads to those we have worked hard to evict."

I felt a strong compulsion to share a personal story with Mr. Williams. I asked his permission. "Can I share something with you from my own experience," I asked him? There is always the risk of backfiring when the counselor shares personal information with the counselee. It's rarely professional, I admit.

I shared David's story. "One day, my friend David asked if he could speak with me in private,"

"Of course," I responded.

"About six months ago, my father died," David continued. "Yes, I miss him, but I am troubled with his death. He and I have been estranged for a long time. It was about different principles. I wanted to go to graduate school and enter the ministry. He wanted me to follow in his footsteps and go to the Military Academy. We had different values and could never resolve them and stopped trying after a while. I had not spoken with him up to his death. Now I can't talk with him, and there will never be reconciliation. I feel terrible. "

I asked Mr. Williams if he could identify with the story

"That's obvious," was his reply. "So, you're saying there are times when we need to give up our principles, our values for the sake of our relationship."

"I think it happens a lot. People can be vulnerable, especially the ones we love the most."

A few weeks later, Mr. Williams (he preferred I call him Ted now) confessed that he had contacted his son from whom he felt estranged. He said the conversations were awkward at first; they reminisced of times they went fishing together, periods when they shared model trains, and vacations taken together. As the calls continued, he acknowledged they evolved into confessions; what each was sorry about that had happened between them, feelings of regret; that they both had balked accepting. They mutually acknowledge that absence was no longer necessary.

One week later, before my next scheduled visit, I saw that our nurse had pronounced Ted dead in the morning hospice notes at 6:30 P.M the previous evening.

Chapter 7

Ariel's Story – Desperate Days Ahead

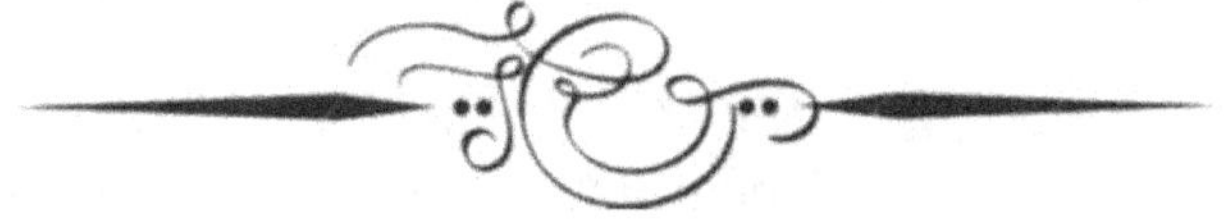

Never allow yourself to be so desperate

that you end up settling for far less than you deserve

- Author Unknown

"Why are you getting up so much at night? I asked Ariel. "Do you feel alright? Can't you sleep?"

"No, not much," she responded. "When I lie on my side, my back hurts so much it wakes me. Walking around for a while stretches it, and it feels better afterward."

Ariel's back pain soon became the focus of our life. It demanded both of us' attention, for Ariel because she was suffering through it and me because it interrupted my daily routine and nighttime sleeping. She didn't dwell on it, at least not by incorporating it in all conversations. Her discomfort dictated, however, how she spent her time during each day. I dwelled on it because I felt not a minute went by each day when I was not seeking some solution to her situation. I felt like it consumed my life more than hers.

Ariel was not sleeping well at night. After a couple of hours, she often woke up, got up, and then wandered about the house occasionally stopping to check her computer or put some dishes away in the cabinets or fold some laundry. At first, I paid little attention and continued sleeping. But as it became more frequent, I sensed her absence in bed. I heard no snoring. She was up and awake in the middle of the night. But why?

Something was changing. No longer did it appear to be just a backache that would heal itself. It now had morphed into something more permanent. I began to question, as did Ariel, the diagnosis of the doctors. Tennis elbow was not sufficient to explain her condition. What were these doctors thinking or not thinking?

Her back should have felt better by now, and it didn't. Ariel continued her work as a hospice nurse without interruption. Never a complaint. Her stoicism impressed me; she became indifferent to her pain, at least on the surface. She kept her feelings to herself. Because she was a nurse extraordinaire, I assumed she knew if it was serious or not. I fully trusted her opinions regarding all things medical. Perhaps because of her easygoing personality, her calmness amid chaos, I accepted her present resignation. If she had only minimal concerns about her back pain, who was I to assume anything different.

And yet, my feelings of confusion and frustration did not fully abate. I assumed the role in our relationship as the "fixer;" the person who found the resources to solve whatever problems needed attention. I believed that it gave me confidence despite any lack of any measure of truth it contained. I am a middle child. I am destined to be the peacemaker who mediates relationships, resolves personal conflicts, and fixes dilemmas. It was only a matter of degree to transpose problems in relationships to problems in circumstances. Right now, the circumstance was that Ariel was in trouble, she had a problem, and I was inept at resolving the situation. This was not as it was supposed to be. Things had to change. But how?

It was early Sunday morning when I got a call from my daughter, Rebecca. "Are you two going to be home this afternoon?" she asked.

"We got nothing on our agenda," I replied. "Why, what's up?"

"Bill and I and the kids want to come down. There are some things we want to talk with you about." They lived about a half-hour away.

"As far as I know, we will be here," I yelled to Ariel in the other room. "Rebecca and Bill and the kids want to come down this afternoon. Okay with you?

"Always like to see them," Ariel answered.

They arrived early that afternoon. Marie brought a friend. She was at the age where she went nowhere without some friend. I hardly ever saw Marie alone when she was not attached by the hip to one friend or another.

In my garage sat two electric scooters. I had inherited them from some friends who thought they were too dangerous for their kids. They didn't look dangerous to me. I suspected they would be fun and entertaining for Marie and her friend. She had mastered the two-wheel bike some time back and showed she was cautious and careful while riding. The scooters handled like bikes, like bikes on steroids.

"I got a couple of electric scooters in the garage," I proclaimed loud enough for Marie and her friend to hear. Her father heard me also. "They are in the garage. Do you two want to try them out?"

"Wait a minute," Bill, her father, interrupted. "I need to check these out before anyone rides them."

Their eyes widened as they gazed at the scooters. "Can we, Dad?" Marie quizzed her father.

We waited for his response as he slowly and cautiously inspected the scooters. He checked the tires, the brake levers, the kickstand, and the brake lights. "You have to wear bike helmets," he stated, which we all took as affirmative to the question of "Can the kids ride them?"

Marie and her friend put on helmets. They were a bit large but functional. Both kids mounted the bikes as if they were "easy riders" and pushed the starter buttons. They acted surprised when the engine started.

Go slow, please," Bill instructed them. It was his final plea as each of them slowly and cautiously moved out of the driveway and headed down the street. I could hear laughing and giggling even over the sound of the motor. They gained confidence, and we saw them turn the corner at the end of the street and disappear.

"I smell trouble already," Bill declared, and we walked back into the house. I was feeling gleeful. The kids' joy took the edge off what I expected would be a more solemn conversation about Ariel's back pain that I assumed was coming.

Ariel was sitting on the couch with Rebecca. Bill and I sat down alongside them. I hesitated to generate a conversation immediately. With some reluctance, I said, "So…. what's on your minds? Why did you want to come down here today specifically?"

Rebecca looked at Bill and then back at Ariel. She took a long, deep breath. "We want to know more about your back pain. I know you are hurting, and we want to know all of what is happening. We want to be helpful, so we need to know everything so that we can support you."

Ariel and I sat quietly for a few seconds. "Mom is hurting," I interjected. "She doesn't like to admit it, but something is drastically wrong with her back. The doctors have not been helpful."

"Have you reviewed with the doctors all the information?" Rebecca asked. "I mean do the doctors know what meds you take and what side effects they cause?"

"They offer no real diagnosis, I stated. Nobody, much less the doctors, seem to understand. They even think it might be in her head, and it's not," I stated. I reminded Rebecca that we had done some preliminary investigations of her medications, but nothing thus far appeared to be a culprit.

Rebecca took a deep breath and sighed. "We want to help."

"We want to help as much as we can," Bill interposed. "We don't want you to feel alone with this. If there is something we can do, tell us."

Just at that critical moment in the conversation when all four of us were deep in thought and contemplation concerning Ariel's circumstance, we were interrupted by Marie's friend who came bursting through the door and announced, "Marie has been in an accident." She was stammering, out of breath, and on the verge of crying.

"What do you mean, in an accident?" Bill asked her.

"She got hit by a car on her scooter; no, I mean, she hit the car."

In unison, we all asked, "Where is she?"

"She is over on the next street, around the corner where we were riding."

"How badly is she hurt?" we asked.

"I don't know. I think she has a bloody nose."

Bill jumped up immediately and ran through the garage and out the front driveway. I followed him and saw him running down the street toward the corner where we last saw the two scooters. He disappeared around the corner. Following behind Bill was Marie's friend on her scooter. She turned the corner and disappeared as well.

I stood in the driveway, watching Bill and Marie's friend disappear. I was not sure what to do now. I parked my car alongside the curb in front of our house. I got in and followed where I last saw Bill. I turned the corner and located Bill a little way up the adjacent street.

Marie was sitting on the curb with her face in her hands. She appeared to be crying. The three of us sat down alongside her. When she saw Bill, she became hysterical, crying profusely and talking unintelligibly at the same time.

Bill uncovered her hands. He checked her face for damage and bruises. "The car just ran into me," Marie repeated over and over. "I didn't see it, and I hit it on the front."

The circumstances were becoming more apparent. Directly in front of Marie was the car she hit. The driver was standing next to the car

"I was parked here at the curb," he told us. "I don't think she was looking ahead and just ran right into the front of my car."

Bill was not paying attention to the driver's words; instead, he was examining Marie. She kept weeping. Some blood was on her face and around her mouth. "I think I lost one of my teeth," Marie blurted out. "I can feel it gone with my tongue." I looked in her mouth, and sure enough, one of her front teeth was missing.

"Where did you lose it?" Bill inquired

"You mean in my mouth or on the street? She asked

We could see where it was missing from her mouth but could not locate the missing tooth in the street.

A man standing nearby told us that someone called EMS and they would be here shortly. They arrived, and two men stepped out of the van and came toward us. One of them stooped down to examine Marie. She looked up at him with her bloody face.

"Am I gonna die?" Tears continued to flow.

"No, honey. I don't think so, but we want to check you out. Can you open your mouth for me?"

Marie stopped crying. "Can we go home now?" she asked her dad.

"She looks alright. Nothing serious, but I suggest you get her checked by your dentist, one of the EMS personnel stated.

"My tooth, where is my tooth?" Marie continued to ask. She burst out sobbing again as Bill escorted her to my car. He drove her home while I remained behind. The day was already a calamity. I was determined to find the missing tooth, to regain some confidence in what otherwise was a disastrous day. I got down on my hands and knees and crawled around near the curbside where Marie hit the car. I scrutinized the area but found no tooth.

I remember the feeling of depression that washed over me. Everything came crashing down; Ariel's sickness, Marie's accident, the missing tooth; it seemed that God craped on me, and I was feeling sorry for myself. I wanted to run away, but I didn't. I returned to the house feeling despondent.

During the following week, we learned there would be a waiting period before a dentist could determine if Marie's teeth only needed fixing or if permeant damage occurred. Life appeared to drag on for a few weeks, burdened by Marie's dental concerns combined with continued back pain for Ariel. Nothing was resolved. Having no resolutions was a thorn in my side, an aggravating annoyance about which I could do nothing. It added to my feelings of utter frustration. Not knowing is often more unbearable than bad news. The bad news is fixable; it's a problem to be solved. Not knowing is ambiguous and obscure. It presents no options.

"Why do you continue to work every day when your back causes you so much stress?" I asked Ariel one morning. I was expressing my frustration, not hers. "Why don't you tell them you need to cut back at least some hours?" I hounded her continuously with my concern despite knowing that asking her to give up work was like asking her to relinquish her firstborn child. It was like talking to a bush.

Despite my concerns and anxieties, she continued to work. Because she had always been a nurse, ever since she was twelve, she was not about to quit now. Her tenacity was dogged and difficult for me to comprehend.

"I need to work," was her usual response. "It takes my mind off other things." At home, she spent time pacing the floor and occasionally inputting data in her work computer. She was not able any longer to sit still and complete computer entries at one time. Sitting hurt her back, and lying down was even worse. This was in addition to the many hours she spent on the road visiting patients at home or in nursing facilities.

Sleeping became an issue, both for Ariel and me. Sufficient sleep had always been important to me, a safeguard to my sanity. I assumed it was the same for all people. I thought eight hours was a standard and transferred that standard onto Ariel.

When the back pain altered Ariel's sleep patterns, I felt she was being denied sufficient sleep. I became upset more than she did. I became obsessed and insisted she address this issue.

"You certainly are not sleeping enough," I told her emphatically. I wanted to be correct. "How can you continue likes this – no sleep? You can't work each day without sufficient sleep." I was pissed off because she was disturbing my sleep as well.

"Stop worrying about me," seemed to be her usual mantra to my harangues. She was frustrated by my repeated criticism of her sleep patterns. "You need to think about yourself," she admonished me, "and stop worrying about me."

Ariel's capacity to care about others greatly impressed me; she always had and did so now. Her moral code was exemplary; her ethical anchor was solidly buried. I think she believed that people do not exist for their own benefit; rather, they exist to serve others. It was her only justification for personal existence. She was certainly not a saint but came as close to being one as anyone I had ever encountered. I admit to a biased opinion, but my judgment did not overcome my frustrations with her sickness. It was hard, and at times completely unbelievable, to acknowledge that she was always supporting me in whatever endeavor I was experiencing at the moment when she was under extreme physical duress herself.

Ariel insisted that I sleep well. She told me that I needed to take care of myself so that I could care for her, when and if" she needs that assistance. It was the "when and if" clause that so conflicted me. Rationally I understood that I was to be her primary caretaker, but, at the same time, I was dealing with an inner feeling wishing that she was not sick and life could return to normal, the way it used to be. I was not a happy camper. I bordered on denial.

Chapter 8

Fears about Death and Dying

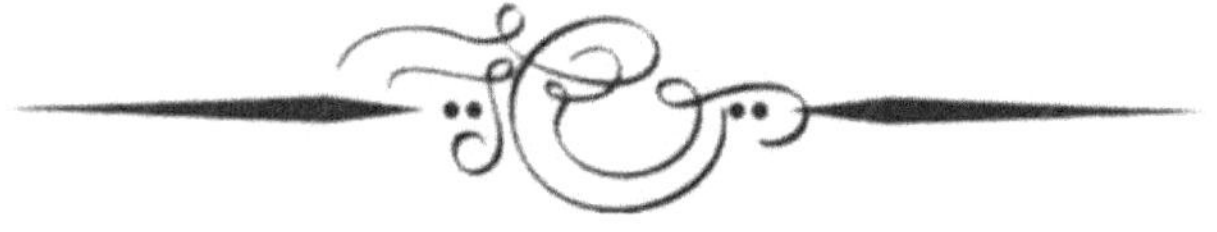

The fear of death follows from the fear of life. A man who lives fully is prepared to die at any time.

- Mark Twain

I have encountered many patients who expressed fears about dying. Those who articulated these fears tended to be extremely frightened at times. I know I am dying," one patient told me. "At first, it frightened me, scared the shit out of me actually, but the longer I lived with this reality, the more I came to accept death as inevitable. It happens eventually to all of us, so why get so bent out of shape."

Others reacted differently. Some patients had no problem admitting to themselves and sharing with their family members' that they are dying. To say "I am dying" without a great deal of anxiety was a positive attribute. If I asked, "is it difficult for you to acknowledge this?" they said no. It bothered them only minimally. I suspect that they prepared themselves; long before they became patients of hospice. They confronted the reality of death and dying in their life, in their terms, and became reconciled with it.

Most patients, with few exceptions, confronted the possibility of their death long before they became patients of hospice. As a condition for hospice, they had to receive a diagnosis of a terminal illness. Six months left to live was mandatory. Many lived beyond the six months, however, and others died prematurely. Either way, they made mental preparations.

The medical community defines palliative care as treating the discomfort, symptoms, and stress of serious illness. It provides relief from distressing symptoms accompanying terminal diseases. By the time hospice admits a patient into care, they have probably, but not always, thoroughly digested the possibility of imminent death. We make it abundantly clear that they are in a hospice program because their medical team decided that there is no cure for what ails them, and their disease renders their life span to six months or less. Many patients far outlive the six months prediction, but few survive the terminal illness altogether. Some folks live in denial throughout the entire period of hospice care.

Palliative care does not mean that hospice advocates dying. But we don't avoid the subject either. In my case, the chaplain's role is to address the spiritual concerns and emotional struggles of those facing terminal diseases. It is often the case that the patient is not afraid of death but is fearful of dying. There is a difference.

People are often afraid to die, but pinpointing what part of death they're scared of can help. Are they afraid of dying alone? Are they afraid of suffering or pain? Are they afraid they'll die, and there will be nothing beyond earthly life? Is there a fear that their lives had no purpose or meaning? Trying to figure out what worries they have can help them face those fears and manage the anxiety. It also allows others to offer support and care for them better.

Mr. White's Story

"I know I am dying," Mr. White told me. "At first, it scared me, really frightened me, almost to the point that I wanted to kill myself. But the longer I lived with this reality, the more I came to accept death as inevitable. My life is not unique. Others, just like me, will die as well. So, I can't act surprised."

Only a few patients of mine were willing to express their deep fears about dying. That is not to say that all the others accepted their fate with joy and eagerness. But for those who articulated fears, these patients tended to experience frightening times. Constant worries plagued them, less so about death itself, but more so about the process of dying.

People fear dying for various reasons. It is the process of dying that they anguish over the most. Some fear dying will involve terrific pain. Since dying comes only once in a lifetime, the fear of the unknown can be overwhelming. No one has prior experience in death. Remaining in control of our lives is vital to most of us. Dying is to give up that control. What we fear is the loss of control.

Having an untreatable terminal disease is a condition for acceptance into hospice. Under most circumstances, by the time a patient enters into a hospice relationship, that person has thoroughly digested the possibility of imminent death. Palliative care then focuses on death's reality, but with a caveat that it does not have to include suffering. Hospice care is comfort care.

Mr. White exemplified all of the above symptoms. The doctors diagnosed Mr.White as being terminal with COPD. When I first visited him, I found him confined to his favorite easy chair in the living room. It was a Barcalounger type chair where he could sit upright with his legs extended straight out in front of him.

"Are you comfortable in this chair?" I asked him

"Depends on what you mean by comfortable. I am never really comfortable, but this chair is the best I can get," Mr. White replied. He was able to shift his weight by pushing his bottom towards the chair's back and scooting backward at the same time. It allowed him to sit more upright.

"My legs feel better when they are straight out in front of me," he remarked as he wiggled his legs into a more relaxed position.

Mr. White told me that he and his wife have lived in this house for the past ten years. It was a modest house he acquired after he retired from the electric company. He spoke proudly of his work as a pole climber.

"Don't have pole climbers anymore," he told me. Now they have mechanical buckets to reach the top wires. Didn't have them in my day. It was all physical climbing."

Mr. White spoke of his strong Christian faith, frankly and forthrightly.

"My wife and I have devoted our lives to our church. We have always been right with God and Jesus. We count on God now to get us through this time. We pray a lot, and our faith is strong."

He then sat for a minute, looking directly at me. "Can I tell you something I have not told anyone else?"

"Of course," I started to prepare myself for some new revelation. I was primed to be surprised.

"My faith has always supported me," he said. "I have no doubts about that. But I have some uncertainties that cause me anxiety. Don't know if it's because of some lack of faith or if it is something else. I always count on my faith to make things right, but I have this fear about what will happen to my wife and family after I'm gone."

I quickly realized that it was not his faith he worried about; rather, it was about his wife and family's well-being due to his death. His faith's strength sustained him personally, but he saw no relationship between his strong faith and his family's welfare—separate considerations with different consequences.

"Have you talked with your wife about these concerns?" I asked him

"A little bit. We talked about fiancés and wills, and advanced directives, and other stuff, but that's all on paper where she can read it. What I fear the most is emotional. Will she ever get over me being gone?"

"It takes some time for people to grieve, but eventually, they can move on," I told him. I immediately sensed this was not what he wanted to hear. He looked away and sighed.

"I told her that she would need to get on with her life and let me go when I go, but I am not sure she is mentally and emotionally capable of doing that. She is much too attached to me, too dependent on me."

"What do you mean too attached to you?"

"I have always been the fixer for her. Whatever goes wrong, I fix it. Not just stuff, but personal problems as well. She grew dependent on me for all things, and I let her because it made me feel important."

"Maybe she is more prepared than you think," I answered. "I thought I told you that she had shared some of these concerns with me on one of my visits while you were sleeping. I think she recognizes that she will miss you a lot but is not as dependent on you as you think."

This revelation came as a surprise to Mr. White. "What do you mean?" he queried.

"What I mean is that we talked about her permitting you to die. She knows that you think she is dependent on you, but she has an independent streak of her own. She lets you think she is dependent because she knows it makes you feel important. She wants you to feel good, but sometimes that feeling gets all mixed up with other feelings."

"Wait a minute." Mr. White interrupted me. "All she wants is to make me feel good?"

"Hang on a second," I told him. "Don't jump to conclusions. I think your wife is trying to say that she wants to permit you to die. Do you know what she means by that?"

"She wants me to die?"

"No, not at all. But if you are going to die, which you are sooner rather than later, and you know that as well as I do, she wants you to know that she will be all right. She has learned what self-sufficiently needs to be after you are gone, and you don't need to worry about her. You can go in peace, in other words."

"What a horrible thing to say to someone you love," Mr. White responded. "It's like telling me she's had enough, and I can just go now."

I don't think that's what she means," I said. Without precisely knowing what she meant, I settled on the following explanation, which I hoped would clarify her motivation for him. I said, "Sometimes the most compassionate act you can take towards another person is to permit them to die. Yes, even if you don't want to lose them. Even if you think you can't live without them. There are times when you have to let them cross over; they need to know it's okay for them to leave. Sometimes they are only waiting for your permission."

I completed my mini discourse but sensed that Mr. White was unimpressed. Maybe he thought it was a diatribe; I was seeking to appease him by using explanations he was unwilling to accept.

"I will have to think about all this," he said.

"Can I come back for another visit, and we can talk more about this," I asked. When I feel I am on shaky ground, I like to postpone to reorganize my thoughts.

I remember a conversation I had with a mentor of mine before assuming responsibility as a spiritual counselor for Hope Hospice. He addressed the issue of preparing to die. "One of the kindest things you can do for another human being," he told me, "is to permit him to die when it is his time to go, and he is suffering. 'There is no need to rail against the dying of the light because what is on the other side is like going home. Don't anchor people's energy here by keeping them on life support for months or years. You're keeping them from peace. It's hard to let go, yes. But remember that they are not going anywhere. They are just sloughing off their physical shell. They are intact and whole on the other side. Honor those you love by releasing the emotional tether that holds them to earth. Honor those you love by permitting them to let go and cross over. Let them know they have nothing to fear, and you will be fine without them. Tell them you will miss them, but fine despite their going away. Let go and let God."

The fear of death is quite common. People fear death in varying degrees. Some fear their death while others fear the death of someone they love, someone they feel they can't live without. To what extent the fear appears and in what context it happens varies from person to person and circumstance to circumstance.

During my tenure as a hospice chaplain, I have observed different patients with personal fears about dying, but not always for the same reason. Some fears are about pain and suffering. Others, when they are close to dying, fear they will experience excruciating pain. One patient who was in "transition" (That period when the medical community indicates death will occur momentarily) while I was present, but still had a sense of consciousness, told me," My heart is racing. I feel sharp pains in my chest. The room appears to be spinning out of control. I don't know what's going on, but I know that something terrible is happening. It feels like it may be a heart attack. I feel a sense of doom, as though the world is about to end." Strange illusions, but real to the patient.

"Do you have any feelings about what happens to you after you pass on?" I once asked a different dying patient. "I am afraid of what I don't know," he responded. Fear of the unknown; what happens after death remains a secret, and it is human nature to be bothered by what they don't know. It is not unusual, nor is it a psychological block to fear that death is final. People who have read existential philosophy (Sartre, in particular) are particularly susceptible to fear the unknown that accompanies impending death. There is nothing more after death.

The Christian faith speaks of death as "entering another dimension." After this life, one passes onto another life; eternal life. According to Christianity, each person possesses a soul that leaves a person's body at death and goes to an afterlife in heaven or possibly hell. A reunification takes place, and the recently departed are re-connected with already departed loved ones. These beliefs have a calming and robust appeal to persons who hold their faith firmly. Yet I have encountered evangelical Christians who say they are dubious concerning the afterlife; it might not be real after all. The fear of non-existence still plagues them.

These are common fears for those facing imminent death. Fear of death is not limited to the dying person; it can also plague the left-behind family members or friends. Their worries are less about the dying person and more about themselves; how they will survive without that person.

Martha's Story

Our new patient was a ninety-four-year-old lady with strong Catholic religious beliefs. We assigned our Catholic chaplain, Anna, who attempted to visit.

"They don't want me to visit," she told me one morning.

"What's the problem?"

"Couple of things, the best I can understand. The sisters can't handle a female chaplain for starters, and they prefer an ordained priest, which I am not."

"We're supposed to provide chaplain services," I reminded her. "So, what do you think we should do? Do they want spiritual counseling at all?"

"I called their local priest. He's willing to stop by for the sacraments, but he can't see them regularly as we do. How about you? You're ordained, and you're a male?"

"But I am Protestant, and they are Catholic. Do you think that's a problem?"

"I don't know, "she responded. "But if you are willing to give them a call, we can find out."

It is the mandate of the hospice program to provide spiritual counseling to all our patients. From the outset, we ask if they want a chaplain to visit. One is assigned unless the patient or family flatly declines.

"Hello. My name is Reverend Peter Olsen, and I work as a counselor for Hope Hospice." I was calling from my "office" in the men's bathroom. I often used the bathroom when I felt unsure about addressing a problem patient I suspected was suspicious about having a chaplain. My goal was to convince them that I should visit, but doing so sometimes required some embellishment when introducing myself. I told the truth about being a "reverend" but exaggerated a bit about being a counselor. Other staff members could not hear me in the bathroom.

"We want to be as helpful and comforting as possible for your mother," I told the daughter, who answered the phone. "I would like to come by to meet her and talk with you all about how we can help keep her comfortable." A little embellishment goes a long way. She invited me to visit on Thursday morning at 10:00. Then she added, "Mama's not always awake, and we don't want to wake her if she is sleeping."

"I understand and will be respectful."

I arrived at the home at 10:00 A.M. It was a modest home located in a primarily Hispanic neighborhood. On nearby mailboxes, I could see Spanish surnames printed on them. The neighborhood displayed statues of Mary, the mother of Jesus, a variety of busts of Saints, and an occasional outdoor altar. These folks took their Catholic faith seriously, I thought.

When I knocked on the door, a middle-aged woman dressed in a housecoat and wearing slippers peeked out. "Yes, can I help you?" she said. She looked at me as if I were an unwanted salesman or an intruder who was bent on doing her harm.

"I'm Reverend Olsen from hospice," I told her through the crack in the door. She then opened the door wider.

"Okay, come in. Mama is in the bedroom. She is awake, but I don't know for how long." As we walked through the house, I noticed three other women about the same age sitting in the living room, each dressed similarly to the first woman. I acknowledged them by introducing myself. They offered no response, just stared.

"Those are my sisters," she told me." My name is Martha. I'm the oldest and live here with Mama. My sisters live nearby but stop by to help with Mama."

Mrs. Espinoza was awake in her bed when we got to the bedroom. She looked emaciated. Her arms were extremely skinny, her eyes were open but only as tiny slits, her hair scraggly, and no lips to be seen.

"Mama, Mama, this is Reverend Olsen. He's a priest. He wants to pray with you. Mama, do you hear me?"

Mama looked at Martha, then at me, and back again at Martha. She revealed a slight smile through her pursed lips. I then knew she understood. I said a prayer.

I remained for a visit well over an hour, just sitting by the side of the bed. She never spoke up, but her breathing reflected a comfortable demeanor. There was no apparent crisis at the moment. I watched the four sisters as they catered to Mama, checking on her every few minutes, talking among themselves about what she might need. I learned quickly that there was a strong attachment between the sisters and their mother. They adored her almost as if she were a saint to whom they constantly provided veneration. While listening to their conversations, I heard how much they thought she sacrificed for them while growing up, how, as the family's matriarch, she guided them through rough times, and that they would never abandon her under any circumstances. One of the sisters stayed by Mama's side twenty-four seven. It was Martha, the oldest sister.

My initial reaction was one of admiration and wonder. How awesome it was to be in the presence of a family so devoted to caretaking each other. It was not unusual for a daughter to care for her aging mother, but to encounter a whole flock of daughters providing such care twenty-four hours each day was truly rare. Outside of this family, I never encountered it. I admired the perseverance, particularly Martha's, the oldest, who was constantly present.

As I observed the sisters more closely, a different perspective began to emerge. The level of adoration seemed beyond reasonable. Yes, caretaking demands a degree of attention. Still, the attention given by these sisters went beyond meeting the needs of Mama and bordered more of meeting the needs of the caretakers. The adulation heaped upon Mama and the devotion that was given to her appeared to become competitive among the daughters. Each sister attempted to provide care beyond what the other sisters did, almost as if to say, "I love her the most, more than the rest of you." Each sister tried to surpass the efforts of the other sisters.

Caregiving became compulsive. Tasks were performed despite any necessity. Mama, due to her condition, needed little nourishment. Too much food too quickly caused her to choke. While I was there, one sister brought in food from a casserole on a dish that she piled high with gravy, enough for at least three people. Shortly afterward, another sister had baked a cake and cut a piece at least six inches wide for Mama. Needless to say, she was not able to eat any of it. However, the sisters took turns preparing elaborate meals, each more extensive and more ostentatious than the previous one. The sisters used food as a means of showing love despite that Mama could not consume it. But the sister who provided the best food could claim that she loved Mama the most.

Martha demanded of herself that she spend nights, all night long, at Mama's bedside whether it was required or not. Usually, it was not. Mama slept through the night without complications. Martha's constant residency at Mama's side seemed compulsive; it met Martha's need more than it met Mama's need.

Over two months, I observed this routine regularly. Martha, and at times, one of the sisters, sat with Mama consistently. When Mama awoke, she acted oblivious to the presence of the daughters. She did not communicate with them. I did notice an occasional stare by Mama at one or another of the daughters but without any recognition in her eyes.

The weekend nurse who visited predicted that Mama would expire by the end of the following week. Mama continued to get weaker, ate less food, and stopped taking fluids. No one lives beyond a week or so on such limited nourishment. The nurse reported her as "active" in her report, stating she was in the throes of dying. Early Wednesday morning, the office nurse received a call from one of the sisters who reported that Mama had died.

"When did this happen?" the nurse asked

"Last night around ten o'clock," the sister responded.

The nurse noted that it had been about 10-12 hours since Mama had died, and Mama was still lying there in her bed. Not the usual sequence. When they initially enroll in hospice, the staff asks families to notify our office 24/7 when the patient expires. The morning nurse left immediately to tend to the declaration of death and asked if I would meet her there.

When we arrived, we met one of the sisters, who ushered us into the bedroom where Mama lay surrounded by the rest of the sisters and cousins and nieces. Martha was lying on the bed with her mother. I pulled aside one of the sisters. "Has anyone called the funeral director?" I asked.

"No," she said. "Martha does not want to do that."

"What do you mean Martha does not want to do that."

"Martha does not want to let Mama go, at least not yet."

Martha was lying face down on the bed, holding Mama in her arms and sobbing unceasingly.

"Mama, please don't go?" she repeated over and over. Her sisters approached her and asked that she get up. "Martha was closest to Mama," she told me." She just won't let her go."

I watched as Martha constantly wiped Mama's face and neck with a cloth, kissed her on her forehead while holding her head tightly, and caressed her face with her hands. Her devotion was more than compassionate; it appeared compulsive and obsessive.

A half-hour went by and then a full hour, and Martha continued to lay with her mother, hugging her body while nearly smothering her on the bed. She continued weeping uncontrollably. Again, her sisters attempted to persuade Martha to get off the bed and let go of Mama. Martha ignored their pleas.

Shortly after that, the funeral director arrived, prepared to take the body to the funeral home. Martha was either unaware of or chose to ignore the presence of the funeral director. She persisted in her efforts to hold on to her mother, refusing to get off. Despite the gracious words of comfort her sisters or me provided, Martha could not be pried from her mother's bed. She enfolded her in her arms. If Mama was still alive, she would have been suffocated to death.

The funeral director cornered me. "We can't stay here much longer," he said. "I have to be available this afternoon for another death." He pointed at Martha. "She needs to let us take the body."

Again, I tried to reassure Martha. "Martha, the funeral director needs to attend to your mother. I know it's hard to let her go, but she will be in a better place. No more suffering. Let her go and be with God."

"No, no, no." she insisted as she spoke through her tears and sobs. She hung on all the tighter.

I conferred with the sisters. Their husbands had arrived at the house by now. The three husbands decided they would attempt to extract Martha and, if necessary, force her off the bed, despite Marth's protestations. While speaking words of consolation and solace, the three husbands gently but firmly pried Martha from the bed and placed her in a chair nearby. All the while, Martha protested and continued to wail, "no, no, please don't take Mama. She can't leave us."

Two of the husbands stood guard. Martha continued her wailing and sobbing, calling out, "Mama, don't leave us." They attempted to move Martha to another room while the funeral director placed Mama on a gurney and covered her with a shroud. Just as the Director wheeled Mama toward the door, Martha broke free, grabbed the side of the gurney, and attempted to throw herself on top. The husbands thwarted her while Martha shouted, "Please, Mama, don't leave me."

The sisters were able to escort Martha into another room. I met with them all and shared a prayer of release, asking God to take Mama into his arms and give her peace and bring healing to this family.

How people react to the death of a loved one vacillates greatly from indifference and apathy to overreaction and downright melodrama. Neither is improper, or without deference; instead, they are just dissimilar responses to the same experience. I experienced some families who are truly relieved when a loved one passes. And I meet others who forever regret the day that death took their loved one. We cannot be judgmental about any of the motivations or circumstances. The realities of caregiving can be stressful and demanding. Fears related to dying express themselves openly and frankly; they harbor deeply held beliefs that are sometimes expressed reluctantly and grudgingly and at other times without hesitation and great passion. Such feelings, either way, are the beginning of the grieving process.

Chapter 9

Ariel's Story - Acupuncture, Arthritis, and Dr. Payne

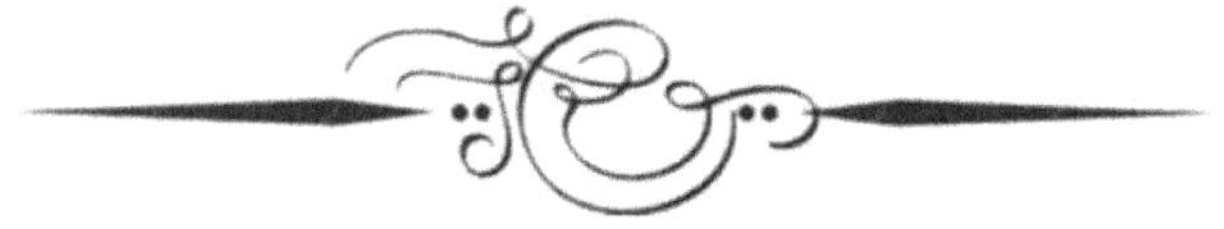

"Some days are better; some days are worse.

Look for the blessing instead of the curse.

Be positive, stay strong, and get enough rest.

You can't do it all, but you can do your best."

— Doe Zantamata

"If I can just get some relief from these back pains, I could think more clearly," Ariel announced one evening as we ate our diner together.

Now that I had retired, I wanted to make meal preparations more my responsibility. I started by making the salads each evening, waiting for Ariel to get home, and "allowed" her to complete the meal. I always felt as if dinner preparation was her job, and she liked it that way. She didn't acknowledge my contribution to be as important as I did and certainly did not admit that cooking was "women's work," but she did express her appreciation for the effort. My retirement needed some getting used to and required some changes in daily routines, at least for me. At first, there were times when I felt put upon or taken advantage of just because I no longer had a "real" job, but Ariel quickly and adamantly put those thoughts to rest.

Ariel had reached a certain level of pain where she no longer refused to acknowledge it. She now admitted she was hurting. She confessed one day, "It's hurting now more than ever," she told me. "I need some relief from this aching."

It wasn't a pain, she insisted. It was an ache in her back, but it ached constantly. I really couldn't see the difference. It hurt her, and that was the important thing. Regardless of her terminology, I supposed that she had reached an intolerable stage. She had pretty much exhausted over-the-counter medications, which she studiously avoided as much as possible. She had experimented with the ordinary Nsaids, pain patches, and hot water treatments with minimal results. She found she needed increased levels of medications to achieve the same level of relief. Her upward spiral of drugs, however, offered no upward degree of comfort.

In between bites of dinner, Ariel interjected, "I have a friend who does acupuncture. She used to be a nurse at Hope Hospice but now has her practice on the side. I talked with her, and she said perhaps she could help with pain using acupuncture."

"I don't think acupuncture will cure anything," I said.

"No, it doesn't cure anything, just helps to relieve pain," Ariel instructed me. "What harm can it do? She has credibility."

Because Ariel was never one to quickly try new things, I got the impression she was feeling more desperate than I thought. For her to venture toward an ancient Chinese folk medical procedure to relive her pain was an acknowledgment that things were getting worse, perhaps even out of control.

Ariel made her appointment. The practitioner had a small office located downtown. "No, she said, "I don't want you to go with me." I didn't protest.

"How did it go?" I inquired when she returned from acupuncture treatment.

"I don't know yet," was her reply. "Catherine (the practitioner) said it might take a while to feel any results. Right now, I don't feel anything, no relief at all. Maybe just a little bit that could be numbness from the needles or maybe my imagination."

While listening to the tone in her voice, I got the feeling that she had some hope, but only slightly. For the most part, she seemed to feel a bit let down and remorseful.

I wanted this to work. I wanted anything that would work. I was beginning to grow weary over what I thought was a temporary setback taking too long to correct itself. My impatience with sickness was starting to emerge again. Unfortunately, despite my resistance to resentment, it was happening nonetheless. We waited a few more days. Nothing changed.

I noticed that Ariel returned to her former position – leaning to the left, not able to stand straight up, holding her arm across her stomach, grimacing. We both lost hope in acupuncture.

Unit now, neither of my two daughters was made aware of the degree of Ariel's distress. Kimberly, the older one, was presently traveling through Asia, particularly in Egypt. Communicating with her was limited. The younger daughter, Rebecca, was married and had children. She knew about Ariel's backaches, but not that they were severe. Ariel insisted on not bothering them; they had their own lives to live, she maintained.

However, it proved impossible for them to remain uninformed. If Ariel was unwilling to reveal her situation, I had no hesitancy to do so, much to Ariel's chagrin. Both daughters stepped in aggressively when informed by me. They each began to explore all avenues where they thought there might be information pertinent to Ariel's situation. The causes of her pain remained a mystery that challenged the two kids. We started a search for potential causes of, and probable remedies for, Ariel's back pain. None of us had any medical background other than pure inquisitiveness and the internet. We did have persistence on our side.

"Let's use the words 'lower back pain' as our search engine," Rebecca suggested. "If we can't exactly find what we need, maybe we can eliminate the nonessential."

The internet searches revealed many different kinds of lower back pains. Unfortunately, they used medical terms beyond our ability to comprehend. Consequently, we had to undertake a brief but comprehensive cursory exploration of medical terms. Still, we wallowed in the dark and felt we exceeded the extent of our pay scales.

Muscular and ligament strain seemed to be the most common causes. These were associated with people who had existing maladies or weaknesses that allowed back sprains to accumulate quickly. These maladies did not fit Ariel's pain patterns. Likewise, arthritis was a common source of back pain. We thought we made a significant discovery here, but it turned out that we were more impressed by the name than by the diagnosis. We eliminated Arthritis as a cause.

When she returned home, Kimberly discovered a disease that none of us had heard of but sounded cultured – Aortic Aneurysm. An aneurysm is a type of ballooning of the aorta running through the abdomen. We were excited; it sounded like we were narrowing on a significant option, an avenue worth pursuing. This type of aneurysm can cause substantial pain extending from the belly button and continuing straight back, depending on the type of aneurysm. Since Ariel indicated that her pain was not solely confined to her back, but instead surrounded her midriff area, perhaps we were on to something significant. Unfortunately, time and further investigation proved we were wrong again. If it weren't for bad luck, we'd have no luck at all.

Fosamax was the next culprit we explored. Ariel was prescribed this medicine for osteoporosis relief and prevention. Internet sites indicated that Fosamax caused bone loss in the jaw, among other facial symptoms in some cases. Of importance to us was the revelation that Fosamax, on occasion, contributed to burning pain under the ribs as well as in the back and abdomen. This was precisely where Ariel identified the location of her pain.

We became elated, not because of *her* pain, but because we found a cause for her pain – Fosamax. The company that manufactured the medicine already had many lawsuits filed against it, and we decided that one more was not going to bring relief to Ariel. Besides, further research cast considerable doubt on any Fosamax effects that might have caused Ariel's situation. Another dead end.

We researched pain patches. Ariel had tried many and most offered little relief. Then her physician suggested something new – physical therapy. It sounded ridiculous, but what the hell, who were we to judge. Anything was worth a try.

I went with Ariel to her first session of PT. It was agony to watch. She rolled across mats set at different angles, hung by her arms from railings above her, and was twisted into various pretzel shapes, all to relieve pain. The "healing therapy" only caused further pain and distress. Still, not a word of complaint from Ariel.

Desperation began to set in. I felt at a crossroads. Ariel's pain was constant; no respite in sight. Frustrations settled in with me. I grew impatient. I tried to keep those feelings personal, but an outburst would erupt once in a while, and I would infer blame on Ariel for being sick. I acted so unfair and with such a lack of empathy. My feelings had a life of their own.

Dr. Payne was a doctor of osteopathy (D.O.) who specialized in pain medicine. Pain medicine is a medical specialty that focuses on the evaluation, treatment, and prevention of pain. When our physician suggested we visit Dr. Payne, it sounded like a joke – Dr. Payne, a pain doctor. We scheduled an appointment nonetheless.

Dr. Payne didn't look a day over twenty-five but came highly recommended. He took Ariel on as a patient immediately. I guess he was competent, but I never felt assured of this. I think it was because of his name. Over the next month to six weeks, he prescribed a whole host of pain medications in ascending order of severity, none of which proved effective.

Ariel reacted to these drugs haphazardly. Some offered no relief whatsoever, while others rendered her almost comatose. For example, her reaction to morphine was immediate and drastic, but not necessarily as intended. It did little to relieve her symptoms but did cause considerable bodily dysfunction. She sat on the couch with a blank stare on her face and mumbled incoherently.

"Do you feel any relief from the pain?" I asked.

"It took her a moment to respond, "What?"

I repeated the question.

"No, it hurts still (mumbling)

"Do you know where you are?" I asked

"Uh…. What do you want?" she replied.

Her eyes drooped as if she were about to fall asleep, yet all the while remaining semi-conscious and awake. She desperately said she wanted to sleep, but if it happened at all, it was only temporary, a few minutes or so, and then she awoke again. She would get up, not sure of the place or time of day, and wander about the house, picking up clothes, putting dishes in the sink, gazing at her open laptop. It was as if she was sleepwalking until the morphine wore off. As far as I could tell, the medications served no purpose for Ariel. When regaining alertness, she claimed she was fine, but clearly, she was not fine.

This see-sawing between medications served no purpose. Despite regular appointments with Dr. Payne, no new information or diagnosis emerged. I suspected that Ariel presented an enigma to the good doctor. I think he gave us his best remedial medication acknowledgment but still unable to offer significant respite. I suspect that Dr. Payne entertained thoughts that Ariel's sickness was at least as much psychosomatic as it was physical. Still no progress and another dead end. The depression and disappointment I was feeling only increased as a result of seeing no solutions. Would this never end?

What comes next was our biggest concern now. Where do we turn for help? Moving on with new or additional physicians seemed to be the only option. To do nothing was not a consideration. Second or third medical opinions seemed logical when first opinions proved insufficient or exhausted. Someone recommended an excellent rheumatologist. Why not? When grasping for straws, you try everything. We had no real reason to go to this doctor, but then again, we had no reason not to go—any port in a storm.

"We need to run some tests" were the first words uttered during our initial meeting with the rheumatologist. I wondered if it was mandatory that all doctors "run tests" before talking with you. While waiting for the test results and X-rays to come back, we reviewed Ariel's plethora of medications. "That's a lot," was the doctor's "visionary" response. We reviewed previous physician diagnoses such as "tennis elbow" and "psychosomatic." It took great restrain on my part to keep from bad-mouthing previous doctors for fear that they might all be colleagues and in cahoots together.

"You need to be careful what you say," Ariel reminded me.

"But I get so upset at the audacity and arrogance of some doctors who seem less intent on living up to their medical responsibilities and more intent on collecting their fees. They don't listen. You tell them what you are experiencing; it goes in one ear and out the other. It sounds as if you have no medical degree; you are not entitled to have an opinion."

"Calm down," Ariel told me.

I settled down begrudgingly. After more conversation with this doctor, I realized she was welcoming and empathic toward Ariel. She listened. She paid attention when we talked. She showed compassion. She sent us home with no new knowledge but with an assurance that she would do everything she could once she examined the tests and x-rays more carefully. She made us feel good. She gave us some hope.

One week later, we scheduled a return appointment with the rheumatologist. "I can go alone," Ariel insisted. I knew that what she meant was not to cause me any additional annoyance. I suspect that she was aware of my unhealthy frustration. I was bad at hiding my feelings. It was in her DNA to consider other people first. I tried reasoning with her.

"You have too much medication in your system. I don't trust your driving," I said. She took offense.

"I am not an invalid," she stated emphatically. "At least not yet."

I insisted on accompanying her and driving, much to her dismay. She hardly said a word to me for the duration of the trip.

"I see nothing unusual," the doctor remarked. We all stood in her office staring at the x-rays projected on the wall. To me, it looked like a menagerie of lines and shadows. "Nothing of note," she repeated. "I'm sorry, but I cannot see anything that would cause your pain."

Not to be deterred, Ariel blurted out, "I can show you where the pain is." She swept her arms around her belly. "It just radiates around my midsection. I can't understand why you can't find a cause?" She burst into tears. I hugged her tightly but said nothing. I could feel her desperation. She was telling us not only that she hurt physically but that she was feeling abandoned as well. I thought that she was about to give up and accept that she was dying.

Chapter 10

Permission to Die

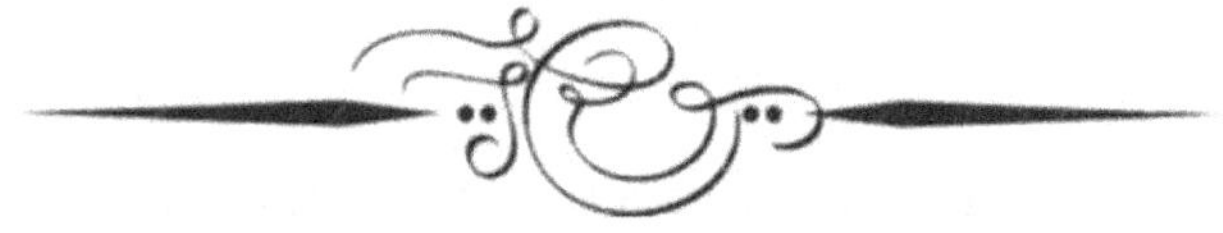

"Another heart attack catches me before I've fallen

I see my life before my eyes and it's soon forgotten

I wanted less to do with it; you wanted it all down baby

I cut the strings and watched you fall, that's all

This self-made soul has gone on too long

I've been waiting permission to die...

But it's just no good for me

Set me free and leave me alone."

Permission to Die, lyric's

- By James Christian, Jim Bell.

Our culture tells us we should fight hard against age, illness, and death, especially death. The poet Dylan Thomas reminds us, "Do not go gently into that good night." Holding on to life, to our loved ones, is indeed a basic human instinct. However, as death approaches, which it inevitably will for all people, "raging against the dying light" often causes unnecessary and additional suffering, and "letting go" might instead be the best option.

One of the greatest gifts we can offer our family and friends is helping them to die well. Sometimes they are ready to go; they know it, but we have a hard time letting them depart. We have to learn to sit quietly with them and utter words like:

"Do not be afraid....I love you....It's time for you to go in peace....I won't cling to you any longer...I set you free....Go gently now. It is the greatest gift love can give."

Henri Nouwen.

The idea that a dying person is waiting for permission to die seems absurd. I suspect it's true that some patients may linger because they worry about the ones remaining behind. Consider this. How do we know it is okay to go? Have you died before? Do you know how it feels? No, you don't- none of us do. Dying is scary stuff even for patients who have strong beliefs in the afterlife.

What if the patient has had enough of this life and feels he/she has earned the right to die, to end it all now? Some people earnestly believe there is a better place than this ethereal world. These are questions people have asked themselves. The Christian believes that life is "borrowed" to be returned to God when our time is up. Who decides when our time is up –only God? Never forget the power of letting go. Likewise, never forget the price of holding on too long. Many families beg the terminally ill to hang on; try one more treatment, try to stay alive if not for you than for us. "Do it for me."

Hang on, but at what cost? Another life-sapping round of chemotherapy? An extra month of pain and suffering? Having to force down food that has no taste and upsets the stomach? Is it worth it?

As death nears, a person might feel a lessening of their desire to live longer. This feeling is different from depression or thoughts of suicide; rather, it's just a feeling that it is time to let go without fear. Some people describe it as profound tiredness that does not go away with rest. Refusing to let go can become more time for suffering than for love.

Family members may experience a change also. At first, they adjust to managing the chronic illness but soon learn to accept the inevitability of death. Finally, as the patient sees, they may see that dying is the better of the two choices. That's when permission to die becomes a mandate. Consent can relieve the patient's distress. It is an act of kindness to say, "You may go when you feel it is time."

These are a few of the thoughts and considerations that terminally ill patients and families have to consider as they face death together. I share with you what others have shared with me. It is always in the context of "permitting to die" that the hospice chaplain attempts to minister to the terminally ill patient and the family.

Mr. Hodges Story

When I first met Mr. Hodges, a hospice patient suffering from COPD, I was impressed by his "take charge" attitude. I say "suffering" because this disease rendered him barely able to breathe. Typical symptoms of COPD include, but are not limited to, shortness of breath, wheezing and chronic cough. Atypical to Mr. Hodges was extreme exhaustion and generalized fatigue. Not all who experience COPD are necessarily so despondent. He acknowledged being on the cusp of imminent death. His sickness had exhausted him.

Many patients with COPD symptoms do continue life for some time but often experience a life full of extremes –Excessive coughing and wheezing, shortness of breath, and severe body weakness. That he was an ex-smoker, still sneaking cigarettes occasionally, only further aggravated his condition. Still, he impressed me as a man in charge of his life and not about to give it up to some silly disease called COPD.

Mr. Hodges, I learned, had been the president of a medium-sized electric company. He estimated he did over a million dollars of business each year. Although he spoke freely and glowingly about his company, he never divulged if he enjoyed the work. Because I thought attitudes toward work experience often give clues to quality-of-life issues, I was anxious to explore this theory despite his hesitation.

So, I asked him directly. "Was the work important to you? Did you like working?"

He studiously avoided a direct answer. "I had responsibilities that I worked on; things that had to get done, and I got them done." A well-designed and evasive response.

My task as chaplain was always to focus on what's most important to the person, especially in the present. I wanted to scrutinize his life, discern his personality, and probe for evidence of what was important to him, whether he was cooperative or not. A person's profession often reveals character; it's a clue to one's satisfaction with life and an indication of the person's inner self-worth. Self-worth reveals spirituality, the primary bailiwick of the chaplain. Being a hospice chaplain, that's the direction I seek, so I plunged onward.

I persisted. "Your company has been successful; I have friends who have bought some of your equipment. Top-quality, they say. Does knowing that reputation make you feel good?" I was phishing.

He avoided a straight answer. "It was tough work to build up a reputation,"

I was not going to our conversation flow on without a response from him. I felt on the verge of breaking through to his more intimate feelings. Again, I asked, "How did you like this kind of work?" I became insistent.

I pursued this stratagem for a while, asking subjective questions while he responded objectively. "Most of the people I employed liked working for me. I think I was fair, and they responded with their loyalty."

Once more, I asked, "What about you? Did you like the work?"

"It was okay." Ah…a little headway, I thought

He remained aloof and was not about to answer my questions in any detail. I got the impression, however, from his description of the loyalty of people who worked for him that he liked being in charge. This loyalty factor gave credence to his self-esteem, but expressing these feelings made him uncomfortable. I realized that pressing the issue might jeopardize his willingness to continue the conversation. I changed direction.

I moved on to other subjects in the slim hope of discovering some inkling of his spirituality. He had previously appeared at ease talking about his family, so I moved in that direction.

"What's most important to you right now," I asked

"My family." I finally got a reply that gave a promise of further exploration. I pursued queries about his family.

"Can you tell me more? What about your family is important now?"

"I worry a lot about them."

"What worries you the most?" I asked him.

"I worry how they will get along without me. I know I am a control freak, and I tend to make all the decisions and don't usually consult my wife. Now I think that is probably a bad trait. That's just the way I have always been, I suppose."

I thought about this conversation for a week or so. On the next visit, I made a point of isolating Mr. Hodge's wife that I might get a sense of her feelings if she was not in the same room as him. I asked her if she thought her husband was a control freak.

"Yes, that's right. Most of the time he *is* in control." She emphasized *most of the time*. "He is not bossy or overbearing. He is certainly not abusive if that's what you mean. He just likes making the decisions, always has done it. He thinks he is the best person to make the decisions."

"No, I didn't mean to imply that he might be abusive," I told her.

"He is a typical alpha male. It's hard for him to stop giving up on that," she responded.

"He tells me that it bothers him. He thinks you might not be able to carry on after he passes. I got the feeling that making all the decisions makes him feel estranged from you and the family at times, like he was the boss of the company."

"Yes, that happens sometimes. But I think we understand him. What can we do?"

In my capacity as a counselor, I have been advised multiple times to shy away from judgments and advice. Listening needs to be my primary focus but in response to the question. "What can we do?" I felt compelled to attempt to answer.

"One of the first things he needs to hear from you is permission to die. He knows he is dying, but like many men, he can't imagine that you are capable of carrying on without him. He needs to hear you say it's okay to go. If you need to go, we will be fine. Don't make it sound like you want him to leave. Just let him know that you all will be fine. You will miss him, but you can move on. You are prepared."

After I had spent time in conversation with Mr. Hodges, his wife called me aside on the next visit.

I have thought about what we talked about last week," she said. "I told him that it's okay to die, but it was so hard, I could hardly get the words out." She was visibly shaking. "It feels like I was abandoning him."

I assured her that it probably was not as difficult for him to hear as it was for her to tell him.

She was not done. She wanted to talk more. She said, "I feel terrible about this, about telling him it's okay to die." She paused for a moment. Her face looked pained, as if she was hurting inside. She looked at the floor, not at me. She then continued, "I sometimes wish he would die soon. It's too hard to wait. I feel so guilty saying that. I shouldn't even think that."

"No, don't feel guilty," I told her when she stood up straight and looked at me. Tears were forming in her eyes. "Feelings have a way of surfacing on their own, uncontrolled by us. You have been through a long, tough struggle with him. It's been as hard for you as it has for him, maybe harder. Sometimes you will feel that you want it all to end and everything to go back to normal. It's not selfish. It's normal?"

When I hear myself dispensing such pearls of wisdom and insight, I wonder if I am serving any purpose other than to listen to my voice. She never responded. She listened, but did not say a word in reply. She walked back into her husband's room.

I encourage patient families to have this conversation with their loved ones. As difficult as it might seem, it can provide natural relief to the patient to know they have permission to let go.

Now and again the most compassionate act you provide the patient is to permit them to die. Yes, even if you don't want to lose them, even if you don't want them to die, even if you think you can't live without them, sometimes you have to let them cross over. And they need to know it's okay for them to leave. They may be waiting for your permission, hoping that you will understand what they need and grant them that wish.

We can choose our time to die if we wish. We know when we're done. But sometimes, people hang on long after they've decided to cross over. Why would they do that? One reason is fear. Many people simply fear death. Some people fear God's judgment. Others who don't believe in an afterlife cling to life because they fear disappearing forever. They fear insignificance, afraid of being inconsequential. No one wants to be a nobody.

Years ago, I helped my mother-in-law decide to cross over. She resisted it for years. She suffered from heart problems and dementia and was living in a nursing home. Her husband was already dead. Her daughter, my wife, also had passed. Despite being told about Ariel's death, her dementia kept her from the recognition of the fact. At night, she and I would have conversations, and I made a point of letting her know it was okay to cross over and that her time in this incarnation had come to an end. She was afraid to let go. She was scared to die. I encouraged her many times, but she just wasn't ready. "Not yet, not now."

Finally, one night she gave me a different answer. She changed her mind. She was ready to go. Three days later, I got word that my mother-in-law died, in her sleep, with no discernible cause. She just slipped away. She joined her husband, Harry on the other side, whole and complete, no longer afraid of suffering.

Honor those you love by releasing the emotional tether that holds them to earth. Honor those you love by permitting them to let go and cross over. Let them know they have nothing to fear and that you'll be just fine without them. You will, in time, join them.

Mr. Roberts Story

Mr. Roberts was not meant to be my patient; I inherited him. He admitted to a predisposition of bias towards female chaplains. He declined visits from Anna.

"Are you sure his name is Robert Roberts?" I asked Joan, the social worker. She had already visited with him and told me that he balked at having a female chaplain, and the supervisory nurse had reassigned him to me. I became his chaplain by default.

"Sounds strange, but that is his name," she responded. A really interesting guy.

"What do you mean, interesting?"

"Give him a call and go visit. Make up your mind. I like him a lot. We've had some interesting conversations. He's not afraid to admit he is an alcoholic."

"Well, I'm gonna take your word here, but if things don't work out, remember I know where you live." For sure, an abstruse response. It felt like I was a substitute for the previous chaplain, not entirely responsible; chaplain by elimination. I might be in beyond my ability. I didn't want to be accountable if the connection deteriorated badly

"He's got a beautiful house, back by the river. Gorgeous spot. And you will love his dog," Joan interjected before she left Mr. Roberts to me

"Can't wait to visit him," I responded. I was still a bit wary about connecting with an alcoholic. My personal bias showed. I was not beyond equating the disease of alcoholism with the ailment of being a drunken derelict.

I read the admission notes for Mr. Roberts. New patients receive an initial evaluation by an admitting nurse. The notes revealed that Mr. Roberts had cirrhosis of his liver, a terminal condition. The cause, probably alcoholism. That was a diagnosis I had not encountered yet. I began wondering how I would respond to a drunk. I reverted to old preconceptions and spontaneously equated the disease of alcoholism with weakness attached to being a derelict, the bottom of the human condition. I was ashamed of myself.

I called Mr. Roberts. I had trouble understanding why a man would have the same first and last name, Robert Roberts. When he answered, I could hardly hear him; he spoke in a quiet and soft voice.

"Hello," he said.

"This is Peter Olsen, one of the chaplains from Hope Hospice."

"Hello, Peter." I think he said. His voice was so low I was not sure I heard him correctly, so I repeated myself. "This is Peter Olsen from Hope Hospice."

'Yea, I hear you. How are you doing, Peter?"

"I'm fine, and you, you doing alright today?" I half expected him to say, "No, I haven't had my quota of booze yet, and I got a miserable hangover." I immediately checked my bias and continued the conversation.

"I know you met the previous chaplain, but she can't visit anymore, and they assigned me to be your counselor. I used the moniker of a counselor, fearful of rejection if known as a religious worker. "I would like to find a time to visit with you. Is there a good time that is convenient for you?"

"Like when?" he asked.

"What's good for you?"

"Anytime. I don't go out anymore. Now is good."

"You mean right now, this morning? "I asked apologetically. I felt my response sounded presumptuous, as if I thought he had nothing better to do than visit with me. "I can be there by 11:00 or so if that's okay?"

"That's good. Do you know where I live?"

"I have my GPS, so it shouldn't be any trouble."

I hung up without saying goodbye. I left the office, got into my car, and inserted the address into my GPS. It told me a time for arrival and pointed me in a direction. I located his home in my GPS on the outskirts of the small village of Wimberley. The social worker said his house overlooked a river. I followed the GPS directions, which always seemed accurate and precise within a few yards of the designated location. I am amazed and confused by how these technical gadgets work.

The GPS directed me toward Fischer, a small village, which I knew was on the opposite side of the river from Wimberley where he supposedly lived. I wondered if I had discovered a hitch in the GPS, a location it could not accurately determine.

My trust in modern technology was unrelenting. The GPS led me off the main road and onto a narrow hard-surfaced dirt road, not much wider than a cow path. There was room for one car. I would have to find a turn-off if confronting another vehicle. The road followed the river for a while and then abruptly turned up a slight hill, then down an embankment and over a low water crossing bridge. These are unique structures in Texas. Instead of situated high above the river, free from flooding, these crossings are only inches above the river. When it rains significantly, the bridge gets covered by the water and becomes impassable. I have not discovered a rationale for why Texas bridges as so constructed. One always takes a risk going across, hoping that rain holds off until after the return trip.

A steep incline greeted me immediately on the opposite side of the low water crossing. The road coursed along a ridge while climbing toward the top and then entered into a wooded area. Still, the GPS urged me onward with the assurance I would find my location only a half-mile further. The road veered to the left, then straight away until it brought me to a sign – 365, the number of Mr. Robert's house. I parked my car.

But there was no house. I did see a pathway through the woods that appeared to lead down toward where I thought the river might be. I walked down the path a few hundred yards and suddenly heard a dog barking. A huge, wooly dog, the size of a wolf, bounded around a corner of the pathway and headed straight towards me. I froze with fear, the kind of fear that feels like you will pee in your pants. My anxiety quickly subsided as the dog started licking my hand while wagging his tail furiously. He was particularly friendly, as he insisted on nudging up to me, so close I had difficulty walking along the path down the hill.

I followed the dog. He seemed to know where to go. I spied the roof of a house closer down toward the river's edge. The pathway led to a porch surrounded by large glass windows, which overlooked a swift-flowing stream about fifty feet below. Across the river were open fields with yellow and blue wildflowers in bloom. The beauty of the place immediately struck me.

The dog announced my arrival by barking frantically at the porch door. A young woman appeared at the door. I introduced myself and told her Mr. Roberts was expecting me. She told me the dog's name was Scout.

"Come in," she said. "I'm Brenda, one of the hospice aides." It constantly amazes me how responsible and conscientious the hospice aides are despite the difficulty of their work and the low pay they receive. "We just finished a bath, and he is in the back room getting dressed." She then moved into the kitchen and started the clothes washing machine. "You haven't met Mr. Roberts yet, have you?" she asked me.

"No, this is my first visit."

"I like him a lot." She continued." We talk about all kinds of stuff. He knows a lot."

The inside of the house was airy and open, with large picture windows surrounding the entire front that looked out toward the contiguous hills. On the back living room walls was a variety of paintings. Some were landscapes I supposed were of the nearby countryside and some that appeared to be modern art. I stood awhile petting Scout, the dog, while I looked at the paintings or out the windows.

"You know I lost this house a few years ago in the big flood." Mr. Roberts stood behind me.

"My first house here completely washed away, and this house is in the same location. I had it built just a year and a half ago. How's that for having confidence?"

Robert looked about in his mid-fifties, but I am not a good judge of people's ages. He dressed neatly in khaki slacks and a cardigan sweater despite the warm weather. He used a walker and shuffled over toward the couch, and sat down with a plop.

"Getting down and up again from this couch is a chore for me now," he told me. "but I'm getting used to it. I like the couch because it is a bit higher and easier to manipulate." He motioned for me to sit in the chair adjacent to the couch. "Sit over here," he said and pointed to the chair. "It's easier for me to hear you when you sit close by." It was more a suggestion than a mandate.

I sat down. The chair was comfortable with extra large cushions. I sat upright rather than slumping back into the cushions.

I suspect Mr. Roberts noticed that and said, "Make yourself comfortable."

Still sitting upright, I said, "I know you had a chaplain before me, but she can't come anymore, so they assigned me."

"Why is that?" he asked.

I hesitated for a second. "I don't know for sure. I think hospice thought I would be a better fit for you. Not all people are comfortable with a female chaplain."

"I like females, no problem there."

"Well…" I felt I had no adequate answer. "It's a crapshoot. We try to match staff with patients the best we can. You just got lucky with me." I felt like I wiggled my way out of that conversation and wanted to move on.

I started to pet Scout while thinking about where I wanted to go next in this conversation. "You sure have a beautiful home here. Great location. How did you find this?"

"I grew up near here and spent my summers camping and swimming on the river. My parents had this land but never built a house here. When I decided to call it quits, it felt natural to come back here. I think I told you this is the second house; the first one swept away in the flood two years ago."

"Well, it certainly is beautiful," I said. "You said you came back here when you decided to quit. What do you mean, you decided to quit?"

"I came back here to retire, I guess. It's not retiring; it's that I got sick and doctors told me I was terminal, that I didn't have much time left. I'm an alcoholic with a heart condition. I still drink and am not figuring on giving it up either. I just can't do that now, so don't go there."

I took that as a warning not to attempt any rehabilitation or preaching. I was surprised at his candor and spontaneity. That he so willingly admitted to being an alcoholic gave me the courage to pursue his life a little deeper.

"How did you get to us, to hospice?" I asked.

"I used to be a teacher in high school back in Princeton, New Jersey. No relation to the university but a lot of our grads went to Princeton eventually. I had to give that up when I got my diagnosis of heart disease. I think I got some liver problems as well. So, I decided to move back here and needed some medical care. My doctor was less than enthusiastic about my chances and suggested I seek out hospice. So now you got me for good or bad. I'm yours."

"You comfortable here?" I asked. "I mean do you have lots of pain or are we helping keep you comfortable?"

He didn't answer immediately. Scout, his enormous lap dog, sat next to me and continuously licked my hand as it rested on the arm of the chair.

He looked at Scout. "I found Scout one day wandering along the river. Don't know where he came from, but since that day and after one big doggy diner, he has never left my side

"Do you live alone?" I asked him.

"No, I got Scout. He doesn't leave me alone. He takes care of me. Let me tell you a quick story about Scout. One time I was watching television. It was an animal show or nature show of some kind. It had a section about snakes and reptiles. There was this one scene about how a rattlesnake warns its prey by rattling before it strikes. The rattle of the tail was loud. Scout heard it and started barking furiously at the television screen as if he was protecting me from the snake. It was surreal."

I noticed how calm and contended he sounded when he talked about his relationship with Scout. He appeared relaxed and without any signs of pain.

"Do you think of Scout as a therapy dog?" I asked.

"Most times, I think of him as a friend, not a dog. I am alone most of the time," he repeated.

I was impressed that Scout was more than just a dog for him. It sounded like a mutual relationship, perhaps the only one he had at the moment. I asked him if he was willing to tell me a little about himself. I felt I needed some background which led up to his decision to become a patient of hospice. I presumed that he was fully aware of his terminal status and that perhaps another human to share his feelings with besides Scout might give him some reprieve and comfort.

Most of our patients have at least a hunch that their time is limited. Dealing with these circumstances by talking often provides some comfort. Robert was on hospice by choice, what feelings did he have about approaching death?

"What's most important to you right now?" I asked. "What do you want to do?"

"I've been living here about two years now, ever since I rebuilt this house after the flood. What do I do? I drink and I think. I'm a tormented man; my own worst enemy, but I don't do anything to improve my lot."

He was on a roll. I encouraged him to continue.

"I have a son who has cancer. He lives in Florida. I worry a lot about him but I don't do anything about it except worry."

"Do you keep in touch with him? Do you want to visit with him?" I asked

"Not really. Sometimes I feel disgusted with myself because I don't want to visit him. I don't do anything for him except worry. I'm good at worrying but not much else. Stay here and worry. Kind of useless, I guess, like I don't care when I do care."

We sat in silence for a few moments. I wondered if Robert felt sorry for himself or just being completely honest and forthright about his feelings. While talking about his son, he showed no particular emotions that I could read.

"Do you have any other family?" I asked as a way to breach the silence.

"I have a sister in Austin."

"You talk with her much?"

"Not much. She comes down here once in a while. She worries a lot about me, but she knows there is nothing she can do at this point. We're close, but I don't make much of an effort to keep in touch. She's the one who makes an effort."

"I don't usually become judgmental, but you sound depressed like you have lost all hope. Do I hear you right?"

"If you mean do I see any future in my life, then no, I don't," he responded.

His contrite response felt like he didn't want to pursue this conversation line further, so I changed the subject. I encouraged him to share some of his past. I discovered we had some things in common. We both had teaching degrees. We both went to boarding schools in New England. We both taught briefly in college.

"Teaching had nothing to do with my drinking," he emphasized. "I loved working with the kids in high school. I never drank or was drunk when teaching."

"Then how did you get started?" I asked. "You mind if I ask?"

"Shit no," he exclaimed. "It's a classic story. Do you remember the movie sometime back called *Animal House*? That's how I got started. I was at Dartmouth College back in the Seventies. Well, my time at Dartmouth was like that movie; parties and drinking all the time, non-stop. During four years at college, I was drunk most of the time, kept drinking long afterward until it became part of my routine, except when teaching kids. Drinking is what I do best now."

His confession's tone did not warrant any judgment or reply from me, so I changed the subject. I felt that I needed to stay away from probing too deeply into his psyche. I feared not being able to handle what might be lingering there.

"Talk to me about spiritual concerns," I asked. I was searching for some content I felt more competent to probe. "You have any religious background that's important to you?"

"Church has never been my thing," he interjected. It sounded at first like a declaration to cut off all communication with the minister, me. I felt the need to respond and clarify.

"I'm not here to preach to you," I responded. "No evangelizing." But it does sound like you got a whole lot of spiritual angst going on, and that must be painful."

Mr. Roberts suddenly got quiet and reflective, perhaps even a little sullen. I thought I had touched a nerve, and he was considering what I had just said. Or, he was about to dismiss me altogether. It was another crapshoot moment.

"I got so many issues I don't know where to start."

Feeling relieved I addressed his response. "Pick a place, any place, and let's start from there," I suggested.

He looked tired. I felt I might still be treading on thin ice if I were to pursue doggedly with questions of a personal nature. I had learned to strike a balance with patients once they began to open up with spiritual concerns, moderating between probing deeply and backing off when the patient appears reluctant.

Mr. Roberts was willing to continue. He shared some back story about his teaching career, emphasizing that drinking was not a part of that experience. He confessed that he was a hopeless alcoholic now, saw no reason not to be at this stage of his terminal disease, and appeared content, knowing that he had little time left to live.

I had been there well over two hours. I decided I had pushed Robert about spiritual issues more than I had intended; any more might sour him on the relationship; I was too aggressive and not to be trusted.

"Can I come back another day?" I asked before preparing to leave.

"Anytime," he stated. And then I left. Scout escorted me to my car.

One week later, I contacted Mr. Roberts, Robert, insisted; I now call him and asked if I could visit. "Anytime," he repeated. On my arrival this time, there was a lady present with him. He introduced me to her as an old and dear friend. She told me she arrived last night and planned to stay a few days. I assumed that there was once, if not now, a romantic relationship between them by the way they bantered with each other.

"If I ever thought about marriage again," Robert said, I would not make a move with consulting Adrienne."

"I can't think of anyone who would want to marry you," she responded. "You are the most preposterous man I ever met. I am the only person who could tolerate you."

"We've been tolerating each other for years," Robert said. "We are attached like Siamese twins."

They spoke of personal times they had spent together and used the word love openly and frequently when describing mutual experiences. The teasing only confirmed my suspicion. I listened for a while until Adrienne interjected.

"Do you mind if I sit in on your visit?"

"I don't," I replied. "But what about you, Robert?"

"No problem. Adrienne pretty much knows about me; more than anyone else. We share thoughts. No secrets here."

Roberts's confession thoroughly convinced me they had a strong personal relationship. I began to consider Adrienne an ally in helping me understand Robert. I hoped that she might also support him and me as we continued to explore his spiritual concerns. Even more important was that she might help convince him to be open about spiritual concerns despite that he might be feeling he has no problems.

"Peter, can I call you Peter," she asked. I nodded yes. "Robert and I have already talked about some of the issues that I feel are important for him to talk about, ones that he tries to avoid as best he can. I may be presuming more than I should, but I feel it would prove helpful if he would share some of these issues, some of his past experiences with you. I might be too close to him. I think you can be more objective."

She looked at Robert. "Am I out of line here?" she asked.

"No. You know me well. I'm open to that," Robert responded.

"What is she talking about?" I asked Robert. "Tell me what she means."

"What she means is that I have a closetful of shit that's hard to open because it's so crowded." He paused for a moment, looking at and petting Scout, who lay next to him. "It's painful when I do it, and it comes pouring out." Again, he stopped talking. He appeared to be ruminating in his mind. He continued petting Scout. "That's why I drink besides the fact that I'm an addict. It takes the pain away."

"Where does the pain come from?"

Robert started fidgeting with his legs. Leg pains were a symptom of his heart condition.

"Tell him, Robert," his friend insisted." Why are you afraid? Talk to him." She turned to me and said, "He needs lots of forgiveness."

I addressed Robert directly. "For stuff that has happened to you or forgiveness you need to give to other people?"

"Both," he said. "But I'm not sure I want to do that. Some of this shit is unforgivable."

"I don't think anything is unforgivable. I don't know how forgiveness works, and I don't know why it works, but I know it works. It's the most tested therapy I know. You can ask for forgiveness from someone else, or you can give forgiveness to another person; maybe even forgive yourself. Either way is hard work but worth the effort. Forgiveness clears the air, gives you room to breathe."

He interrupted me. "But how can you forgive someone who has hurt you so bad that you have never been able to get over it?"

"That's what forgiveness does so well. It helps you get over it," I added. "Tell me more. I'd like to know what's bugging you."

He began to unload. "I was a boy scout. One of the decent things I have ever done besides my teaching." He took a deep breath and let it out slowly. "But what I thought was a safe environment as a kid turned out differently. The scout leader molested me." Again, he paused for a moment. "That so maligned my outlook on life that I never really recovered. I never told my parents. Of course, Adrienne knows. I still carry that shit. I never felt recovered, as they say. How can I forgive him?"

There was a lull in our conversation. I was trying to digest Robert's thoughts and then think about a reaction. Eventually, I got the courage to respond. "He's probably not aware that he needs forgiveness. By now the scout leader doesn't give a shit. But you do. You are still hurting. Forgiveness is not for him; it's for you. You hurt inside because of something that happened, and your anger with him is eating you alive. You got to get rid of that anger, and that's something you can do for yourself despite him. You do the letting go, and you reap the consequences of being free from anger. Otherwise, you remain his prisoner. Don't take that anger to the grave."

Again, we all sat in silence. The intensity of the conversation came to a halt. I felt uncomfortable asking Robert or Adrienne what they were thinking. I also thought for me to talk further would be superfluous. I offered no more. I felt that if I were to press Robert further, he might reject me entirely. Peter, get up and leave the room, I thought to myself. Any opportunity for me to return to continue our conversation might be lost. It was time for me to go. Besides, Scout was barking at the door, wishing to go out.

I started towards the door, intending to thank him for his time and request a return time.

"You don't have to leave now," Robert said.

Adrienne reiterated the feeling. "I think we have made some strides today."

"I appreciate that," I said. "But I have learned that sometimes visits last too long. It's like having dead fish in the house; if they hang around too long, they begin to smell. Best I get going."

A few days before I planned my next visit with Robert, I read a morning hospice report. It said last night Robert passed. A neighbor found him with Scout by his side. The pronouncing nurse indicated he died of "natural causes." However, it crossed my mind that perhaps the conversation we had together mandated a response beyond which he wanted to reveal; it was too exhaustive, too revealing, too personal, and he was not yet ready to handle that. For me, it felt like he chose when to die of his own accord. Nobody, much less any spiritual being, permitted him to do so. He detached himself from his family as if they made little or no difference. I suspect that Mr. Roberts died a broken and lonely man. Of course, this is only speculation.

I had a hard time moving past this experience. I felt I let Robert down, let him drift on by when I should have rescued him. Counseling is the art of allowing the other person peace amid the turmoil.

Chapter 11

Spiritual Heart Attacks

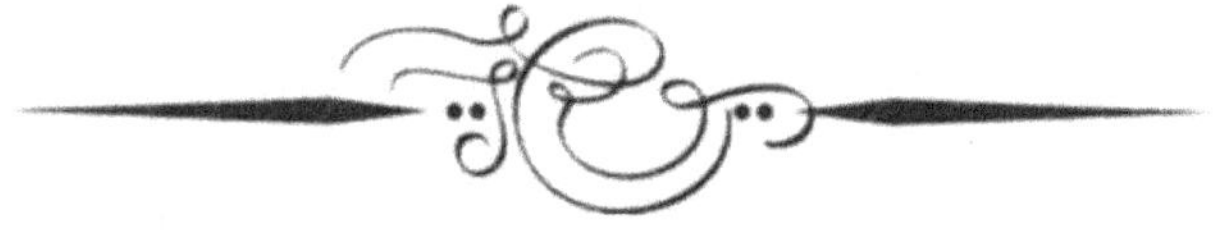

"Victory in the spiritual realm is primary. It is to be obtained by the employment of spiritual weapons."

- Derick Prince

As death approaches, one of the most common experiences I have encountered as a spiritual counselor for hospice patients is the spiritual heart attack. An inherent conflict often occurs between the discipline of medicine and the discipline of the spiritual. The medical field is concerned with the physical and immediate. It focuses on solving the problems presented by the physical body. The spiritual is concerned with beliefs, attitudes, and whatever makes living life essential to the patient.

Spiritually, death is the edge of mystery; death is no problem to be solved. It resists any such explanation. Keeping our attention on the end of life as a "problem to be solved" ignores the end of life's mystery. Addressing the issues of dying without regard for the beliefs of the person who is dying only leads to spiritual heart attacks.

I think spiritual heart attacks are triggered differently for different people. However, there are some common signs and symptoms. One dying woman shared the following attitude with me. "I am tired, and I don't understand why I am still here." Clearly, she was expressing desperation seeing no point in continuing to live. Her loss of interest in life initiated her spiritual heart attack; feelings of anger or depression looming deep in her heart precipitated the attack. Suffering such a personal spiritual heart attack can be devastating. It exhausts all your mental energy and personal resources.

One patient of mine (that you will meet later) directed his anger directly at God. "I am pissed at Jesus," he began. "he doesn't listen to me when I asked him to take me." A misunderstanding initiated this patient's spiritual heart attack. He thought God chooses when and where each person will die, and one merely has to let God know he is ready. If God doesn't respond as expected, the patent becomes irritated and maddened; unreasonable anger torments him till death does him part

A dying person experiences a spiritual heart attack as regret. The person reflected on life and convinced himself that he/she has left undone many important things – "I was a terrible father; I didn't spend as much time with my family as I should have." The person can no longer complete items left undone. He can not heal these wounds and scars. It's too late. The heart was attacked spiritually.

A close second to regret is resentment. Resentments attack the heart spiritually when there is no possibility for reconciliation, or so the dying patient believes. Reconciliation is central to the work of dying. It extends the healing a person can experience beyond one's self to others. Reconciliation is not essentially religious; it occurs in steps: "forgive me; I forgive you; thank you; I love you, and good-bye."

Symptoms of spiritual distress for the dying manifest themselves openly. They can include but are not limited to: feelings of anger, feelings of depression, and feelings of abandonment by God. Besides, there can be questioning the meaning of suffering, asking why I am dying, and sudden doubts about long-held religious beliefs. Certainly not all-inclusive, but rather hints indicating that a spiritual heart attack is about to occur.

When the question is raised about the relationship between physical health and spirituality, medical professional persons often respond, "nothing; there is no connection." These two disciples, science and spirituality, seem worlds apart. Each has a different focus. Physical science focuses on the body, while spirituality focuses on the soul. The physical was the world of physicians, therapists, x-rays, and stethoscopes, a world that could be seen and measured, charted, and analyzed.

On the other hand, we see spirituality as imperceptible, like a breeze blowing through some trees, experienced and unknowable at the same time. The physical was controllable, but the spiritual was only about wishful thinking. Those who think only physically have difficulty once they enter the spiritual realm.

But a person's spirituality is more; it has to do with how he or she makes meaning of what is happening. It affects how a person acts when confronted by adversities. A person's spirituality influences whether we see a disability as an insurmountable barrier or a new challenge. Take, for instance, Mrs. Smith.

Mrs. Smith Story

"Mom says that Jesus comes into her room at night," Mrs. Smith (Sherri)told me on the phone. "She is obsessed with Jesus at her door, and I don't know how to handle her dreams if that is what they are."

I had been visiting with her Mom for about a month. Her severe COPD confined her to her bed without release. She had difficulty breathing and appeared to be frightened each time she experienced shortness of breath. I can only imagine what it might feel like not to be able to breathe. "It's like drowning," some of my other COPD patients told me. Mom was approaching her ninetieth birthday in a few weeks. She complained of exhaustion.

I am tired," she said. "I don't understand why I am still here." For her age, her mind was still active. When she and I were together, we often exchanged thoughts about faith and life, which I found profound. She had an enlightened Christian faith, was lucid about her faith issues, and had extensive biblical knowledge acumen. She particularly liked to recite from memory parables and narratives that Jesus taught. She noted that these narratives exposed the "troublesome teachings of Jesus" because they were filled with contradictions to the ways people usually thought about theological and social issues.

The concern that Sherri Smith shared about her mother was sufficient to warrant a visit from the chaplain even though she did not directly ask me to stop by. I told her I would be there later that morning. When I arrived, she greeted me at the front door and ushered me immediately into the living room. Mom's bedroom was toward the back of the house. The living room was a safe place for her to speak with me about Mom's "dreams," as she referred to them. She did not want Mom to hear our conversation.

"This has been going on for the last week or so," Mrs. Smith told me. "I don't know if she is dreaming or hallucinating, but she continues to tell me that Jesus was at her door last night. I asked her what does Jesus want? What does he say to you? She tells me that's what troubles her; she doesn't know what he wants. I tried to tell her that maybe it was all just a dream, but she gets angry. She believes she saw Jesus at the door."

Is she angry because she doesn't know what Jesus wants or because you don't believe she sees Jesus?" I asked her.

"I don't know what to believe," she responded.

"Let me ask you this. Does Mom seem upset about this experience of Jesus being at her door? Do you think it frightens her? Does she seem scared by these visits?"

"I don't think so, but I really can't tell."

"Let's ask her."

We both went to her room. She was awake and smiled when she saw me.

"Hi, Mom. Do you remember me?" I asked.

"Of course, I do." She replied.

After some small talk about how she was feeling; "fine," she insisted and never mentioned Jesus at her door, I specifically asked, "Tell me about what you see at your door at night."

She looked away for a minute and then turned her head toward me. "Yes, Jesus comes to my door at night."

"You mean you see him standing at the door; that door right there?" I pointed to the doorway between her room and the hallway.

"He is blurry, and I can't see him clearly, but I know he is there watching."

"Mom, are you sure you see Jesus? Do you think maybe you had a dream, and it feels real?" her daughter interjected.

"You think I imagine things, don't you? Well, I do not. I know what I see, and I see him standing by the door, not every night, but most nights." Mom insisted. She sounded a bit perturbed.

"I am sure you do," I interjected. I sensed some conflict arousing and wanted to avoid that. "I think Sherri and I are just wondering what you make of these visits. Are you frightened?"

"Why would I be scared of Jesus?"

"What do you think about these visits then?" I asked her.

"I am not afraid of Jesus. He's my savior. He is here to let me know that I will be with him when my time comes. He makes me feel happy and comfortable."

Sherri and I looked at each other. "Mom feels good about these visits," I said to Sherri. "You do feel good when Jesus visits you at night, don't you?" I addressed the question to Mom. She nodded her head yes.

Sherri left the room, and I stayed with Mom for a while just holding her hand, and shared a prayer with her. What at first felt like a mental health concern, perhaps a spiritual heart attack, evolved instead into a moment of reassurance, a spiritual moment. Mom was not hallucinating, or maybe she was, but it was a moment of spiritual comfort amid impending physical death for her.

For me, it was a case of "whatever works." For the person facing imminent death, rationality is not the most crucial aspect of life; it is not a priority. Determining what is most important to that person at that time and in that place is to enable that person to be in touch with her spiritual soul, the means at hand for bringing that person "home" peacefully.

Mr. Porter's Story

"Can you visit with Mr. Porter?" One of the hospice nurses called me while she sat in her car outside the patient's home. She just completed a visit.

"Yes," I responded. "But Mr. Porter is not one of my patients. I don't know anything about him. Why do you ask?

"I just had a long conversation with his daughter. She told me that he is feeling unusually agitated. Even though his diagnosis is terminal and knows he has little time left, he is constantly complaining about not being able to die. He's impatient. He gets angry quickly, mostly at Jesus, but his agitation carries over towards his daughter and wife. They need some counseling as well as he does.

"Isn't this Mr. Porter who declined chaplain services?" I asked the nurse.

"Yeah, I know, but I think if you go with me at my next visit and we tell him you are a counselor just wanting to meet him, he might be open to a visit. No need to say you are a religious person. The daughter and wife are desperate. His agitation is driving them away, and they don't want that. Besides, he has a loaded gun in the house, which he has said he might use. That's scary."

Suicide discussions are negative warning signs. We take the slightest hint quite seriously. I agreed, and on the next visit, I accompanied the hospice nurse to Mr. Porter's home. His wife and daughter greeted us at the door.

"I told him that you were coming today," she addressed the nurse, "and I also told him that you were bringing a friend, a counselor. He didn't respond, but he didn't object either. That's a positive sign because he objects to most things these days." She then ushered us into the bedroom, where Mr. Porter reclined in his bed.

The nurse took the initiative to introduce me. When told who I was, Mr. Porter looked at me for a moment and then looked away as if to ignore my presence.

I felt I needed to initiate a conversation, or there would not be one. "My name is Peter. I am a friend of Marian, your nurse. She invited me to be here just to get to know you in hopes that we might be able to talk a little about what's happening to you."

After a bit of small talk about how he got to this town from his retirement home in Oregon and a brief introduction to his family background and work life, he surprised me by cutting directly to the chase and opened up about his pain. "I am pissed at Jesus," he began. "I can feel Jesus surrounding my bed. He circles and circles for a while, and then he leaves. I have asked him, prayed to him, that he takes me with him, but he doesn't do that."

I was puzzled. What did he mean, "Jesus is circling his bed?" It almost sounded like he was hallucinating. Not knowing how to respond, I asked him if he could tell me more about this Jesus.

"You know Jesus, don't you?" He sounded annoyed. I acknowledged I did. "I want Jesus to come and take me. I am done living and am just a burden to my wife and daughter. There is no reason for me to be here lying-in bed and having to be taken care of for each little thing. I can't even go to the bathroom myself. My daughter has to help me. Do you know how humiliating and demeaning that is?" He then paused for a minute, turned his head away from me, and muttered the words, *"God damn it."* I could sense his aggravation, an aggravation about which he could do nothing.

Before my visit, the nurse confided in me that Mr. Porter had threatened to take all his pills at once to end his life. He also had a gun in the house that he had access to until his daughter snuck it out of the house. He was not pleased with her interference. These were reasons enough for me to talk with him, to discourage his suicidal tendencies, and offer spiritual comfort.

Mr. Porter was suffering from a spiritual heart attack, a circumstance I had encountered many times while working as a hospice chaplain. His recognition of his physical demise was causing him to reflect on his loss of significance as a person. His spirituality was being challenged, called into question. He regarded himself as a burden to his family, a person no longer with value or worth. When contemplating his future, he saw only a cipher, a nobody.

Consequently, he grew frustrated and angry, foremost with God and Jesus and those close to him; his daughter and wife. He could not accept that death would come when it was ready. Instead, he was insistent that death come when he was ready.

"But Jesus is right here in the room with me," he continually insisted. "I pray that he takes me. I plead with him, but it's as if he pays no attention."

To me, it was becoming clear that it was not the lack of Jesus' response for providing death that bothered Mr. Porter. Instead, it was his feelings of uselessness, his discontent with being a burden to his family, that was almost painful to him. As a self-sufficient individual all his life, a provider to his family, it was inconceivable for him to think of being dependent upon someone else. His spiritual heart attack consisted of suffering the loss of his independence, his most prized spiritual asset.

A second circumstance that Mr. Porter helped me discover concerning the relationship between the physical and the spiritual for terminal patients was that spirituality could make sense of life when the physical structure dissolves. When it comes to our bodies, people rely on healing; they want the experience of being made well again. What people think about when they hear the word "healing" is a cure. They want to be cured of what ails them. They want life to return to the way it was, in other words, to be restored. But there is more to healing than cure. Healing for terminally ill people can also come through coping.

Coping does not mean giving in or acquiescing to a situation. Instead, coping is a means that allows the person to become integrated into the new situation (terminally sick). We can experience healing when we want to return to the way life has previously been. However, when that is not possible, we can still experience a new way of life adapted to the demands of a recent life change. Life is renewed by the spiritual dimension, by learning to cope with what is important to the person at that time and in that place.

A person's spirituality reminds them that life does not end when they can no longer run a marathon or even pick up a dropped book. Spirituality reminds us that something new can still break into our life even as other parts diminish us. Sometimes there is no chance for "cure," and the ability to cope remains distant and impossible to grasp. To those willing to embrace their spirituality, coping can be the saving grace they long for; the motivation to go on despite

Chapter 12

Ariel's Story - The Dreaded Word, Cancer

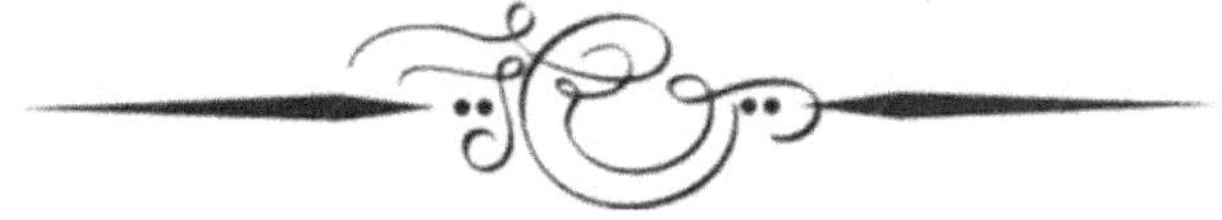

"Your pain is the breaking of the shell that encloses your understanding."

- Khalil Gibran

Ariel decided she no longer was capable of working for hospice. Since the inception of the pain after returning from Disneyland, she had not missed a day for two months. Despite the back pain, the lack of appetite, the absence of sleep, and the medication's effects, Ariel was insistent upon continuing to work. She struggled through each day like a mountain climber intent on reaching the pinnacle despite knowing that she didn't possess sufficient strength. I admired her perseverance but recognized her debilitation. She slowed down to a crawl and eventually stopped working altogether.

Much to her chagrin, her primary physician suggested she get more tests done. Because she felt terrible and had an unexplained disease, he wanted her in the hospital for her tests. Testing in the hospital was less expensive for the patient and a lot less disrupting for the physician. She would have to remain overnight to receive the benefits of inpatient testing. Ariel, of course, balked at this idea but acquiesced after much coercion from the kids and me.

I checked her in one morning, and she was scheduled for her tests that afternoon. Unbeknownst to us, the doctor wanted fluid taken from her chest cavity for examination. Being a nurse, this raised all kinds of red flags for Ariel. The fluid extracted in this manner is only because of suspicion of a severe condition, most likely cancer.

Ariel had a longtime friend who worked in the radiology lab and was a colleague when she worked at the same hospital. She was to administer the procedure. I sat in the waiting room. Hospital waiting rooms have a way of feeling exasperating. It took less than an hour but felt like all afternoon. I fidgeted the entire time, reading all the magazines in the room and talking to other people who wandered past to keep myself from imagining the worst. I admired the dime store art plastered on the walls, typical for a hospital waiting room.

Before Ariel came out of the radiology lab, her friend found me in the waiting area

"We're all done, and Ariel is fine. She will be out in a minute or two, just putting her clothes back on," she told me.

There was a pause for a few moments, and then she said, "We weren't originally sure about this as part of the procedure, but thought it best after reviewing the test results. We had to extract almost a quart of fluid from her chest."

Actually, the doctor suggested this procedure beforehand. It didn't register right away, but I was sure that it was not good news. I surmised that this much fluid should not have been in Ariel's chest by the tone of her voice.

She continued. "It's a good indication that there is cancer there."

That was the first time the word "cancer" was said out loud. Neither of the kids nor I ever suggested that cancer might be a problem. If any of us suspected so, it remained unsaid. Indeed it was on Ariel's mind, but because nothing thus far in her prognosis verified that conclusion, we made no mention of cancer. I did remember when Ariel told me that she would not be around for another Halloween. Cancer as a cause entered my thoughts, but only because it's was a catch-all for people suspected of a terminal disease. The thought was fleeting, however, and not persistent.

They discharged Ariel from the hospital, and I wheeled her out to the car. She so disliked hospitals, outside of working in one, that she stated, "Please don't take me back there again." I acknowledged her request and politely nodded my head as if in agreement.

"Did it bother you when they extracted fluid?" I asked her. Kay, her friend from the radiology lab, accompanied us as we left.

"Not really," Ariel answered. She looked at her friend Kay as if wanting her to answer.

"You're going to be alright," she told Ariel. "I think you'll feel better since we got rid of that stuff from your chest." Kay had tears in her eyes. I figured she was well aware that Ariel had some sort of cancer, just not yet diagnosed what kind.

Ariel didn't speak, just got in the car. "Then she said, "Let's go home, please." I could tell that she was feeling the effects of the cancer announcement. Going home was a return to normalcy, at least for the immediate future.

Today was a turning point. No longer could we deny the seriousness of Ariel's back pain – it was related to cancer. I was unsure how to speak about this. The word, cancer, conjured up feelings of desperation for me as if nothing could make any difference now. We had reached a terminal point beyond which no hope continued. The worst had been spoken, sounding like a death sentence, maybe not today or tomorrow or next week, but it felt inevitable, Ariel was going to die.

Ariel's vitality was beginning to wane; her energy levels dissipated quickly. She no longer felt compelled to accomplish tasks; she resigned herself to become an invalid. Her demeanor changed as well. I thought she was still too tentative to ask for help underneath her bravado, but she now believed that the kids and I needed to take care of her. She was thinking of herself as a burden, an encumbrance, as someone no longer self-sufficient and soon to be a warden of society utterly dependent on others. I had the most challenging task of convincing her that we could take care of her not because we had to but because we wanted to. And yet, I was, at the same time, thinking about all the time and hard work that confronted me and feeling sorry for myself.

I wanted her to feel that she was important to me, that only I was capable of being her caretaker, that I was fully committed to her care, not by default, but by choice. In my heart, I knew this to be both true and false at the same time. There was this constant struggle happening inside me as I felt the commitment to care and the feeling of abandonment at the same time. Long-standing personal ethics and human decency demanded of me that I not abandon her. She needed me. I owed her my best resources out of years of love and respect in our marriage relationship. Yet, that feeling of being cheated out of a future, the resentfulness of having to bear this unwanted burden, was a constant undertone that I could never entirely dismiss.

Chapter 13

Does God Choose When We Die?

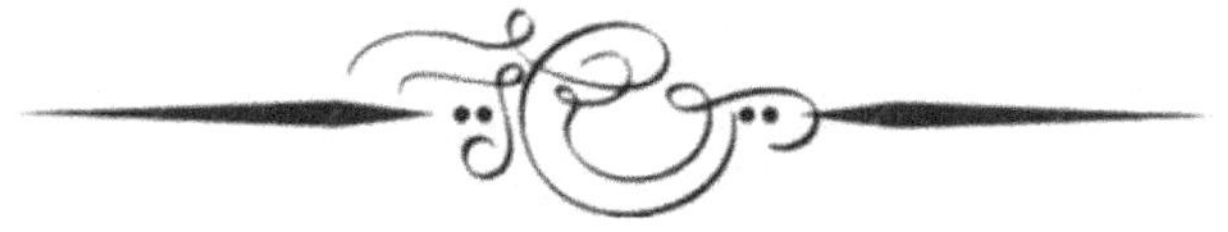

"If the terminal person feels like he is only taking up space and using up resources with no future creativity insight, why doesn't God intervene and end the life?"

- Unknown

Death and dying have a spiritual and religious dimension. People have all kinds of theories about why people die, everything from "they got what they deserved" to "God called them home." All sorts of ideas persist. For some, dying results from a loss to procreate. Still, others consider death as making room for younger people to emerge. There are as many possibilities as there are people who are willing to make predictions. Not all the theories are religiously based or spiritually motivated. Some are outright fantasies, imaginations, and illusions.

Many contend that once a person passes the procreative age, there is no reason to continue to live. God made all creatures solely for reproduction. Others suggest that there is something to accomplish in dying. They are prepared to accomplish "that thing," for instance, the golfer who wants to die immediately after he gets his first hole in one or the mountain climber whose rope broke while scaling the world's highest peak.

Is it normal to fantasize about death? It depends on the person. To some, it appears normal and reasonable, while to others, it can feel like the weirdest thing imaginable. Statistics report that most people do not fantasize about death unless they are depressed sufficiently enough to see life as a burden to avoid.

There is considerable theological thought, however, that death results from a pre-determined date God has chosen. Individuals have no choice; it is strictly determined by "fate." Believing in this fate releases each person from contemplating their demise; thinking about when and where to die is a waste of precious time. God prearranged all things. Why bother to upset yourself when there is nothing you can do about it.

On the other hand, there are plenty of people for whom dying involves choice. At will, one can choose an optimal time and place. Strong feelings accompany one's choice, and people should be allowed to determine this time and place. The reasons for their choice vary from person to person and circumstance to circumstance.

Suicide is one option. People chose to die when they have lost the ability to see a reason to live. Suicide is often a consequence of deep depression, a feeling that nothing makes a difference. Whether they take their own life or participate in some assisted suicide, the motivations remain essentially the same – "I don't want to be alive anymore."

My friend Ron once considered suicide. "I dipped into depression seriously a few years ago," he told me. "I reached the point where I think I was just days away from doing it. Like most people, however, I was too chicken to do it; I was too afraid of the pain of suicide. I'm not brave enough to go through with it. But each day that went by, I was inching closer and closer, and I figured it was only a matter of time. I used to cry, just kill me. I don't want to live anymore." Ron had reason to feel like this. He was diagnosed with testicular cancer.

Ron pulled through, but it was not easy. He relied on his faith in God to help him out of his quandary. He chastised himself and began to think rationally. "Buddy, how have you gotten yourself so lost in the darkness that you can't even see the value of life? If I'm begging God to kill me, it's because I'm ignorant of how much my life is worth, how valuable I am. I'm so lost in the darkness of despair that I believe that that is all there is. That's *wrong*. Not that I am *wrong*, but the circumstance is wrong to live in." Ron recovered.

The idea of taking your own life is a powerful feeling. It almost always is motivated by the same rationale. The person contemplates strong feelings of mental depression, psychotic disorder, a philosophical desire to die, or hopelessness. All of the above have tempted those facing terminal disease. Being terminally sick may trigger thoughts of suicide, but most often, it is accompanied or aggravated by additional impulses.

For many people, this kind of suffering is not a mere allegory; it is as real as pushing against an immovable wall. For them, the pain of living is too intolerable to endure, and the idea of suicide is not an existential, philosophical question or an academic exercise. For these people, suicide is *the only* answer, a way out of misery.

"Deep emotional pain" is a recurring theme in suicide theory, and its debilitating presence has been called the "most common theoretical reason for suicide" The act of suicide is, however, far too complex to sum up in three brief words. Suicides are also extremely rare, and explaining and predicting them can be difficult (Kestenbaum, Robert, *Death, Society*, and Human Existence, 2003, (Routledge: New York and London), 2003,

In his 1952 essay "The Myth of Sisyphus," the French novelist and philosopher Albert Camus wrote of modern man's predicament and described him as an "absurd hero." Man is condemned – like Sisyphus in the Ancient Greek myth – to a life of futility that is devoid of meaning. He must push a heavy stone uphill, only for it to roll back down again once it reaches the top. This labor continues – up and down, up and down – forever. It makes one wonder why this man does not choose to end his suffering? How can such a torturous life be endured?

Camus thinks that man has a noble soul. However, one must possess a certain amount of nobility to struggle against this absurdity of existence. The author believes that life, no matter how seemingly bad it appears, can be lived with a complete "heart" and with dignity. The following folks grappled with these concepts at one time or another in their journeys through hospice care.

Chester Baxter's Story

Chester Baxter died less than one month ago. Silvia, his wife of many years, survived him. She was now living alone in the same condominium they shared for three years before his death.

I went to visit Sylvia. It is hospice policy to follow up with the family of patients after the patient dies. Our program is holistic. We offer services to the whole patient's family after as well as before the patient dies. Family members, particularly the deceased's spouse, sometimes discover a whole host of apprehensions, anxieties, and trepidations that surface following the consciousness and reality of the death.

As soon as I stepped inside her condominium, I sensed that anxiety was consuming Sylvia. After years of observation of patients or church members, I felt comfortable making spontaneous judgments about people's dispositions, especially following a loved one's death. Dealing with death and dying was not a new experience for me. As pastor of local congregations, church members were always dying, and they counted on me to offer condolences and prepare the way toward acceptance.

Sylvia's temperament showed signs of distress. She paced back and forth in the kitchen area, picking up a cup and putting it down again for no apparent reason. She put dishes in the sink and then removed the same plates before she washed them. She jumped from greeting me with a "Hello Peter, how are you?" to "I can't remember who just called me on the phone." Mrs.Baxter somehow connected the two thoughts. At my urging, she eventually sat down in her chair that faced the television, which was not on.

"You seemed to be anxious about something this morning," I commented."

"Oh… I miss Chester so much," she managed to say despite the quivering of her lips. "I just don't know what I will do without him?"

"I understand," I responded, trying to be empathic. "But it has only been a month or so, and you still need time to make adjustments in your life." When I heard myself saying this, it sounded trite and mundane, without an ounce of empathy. My mind harked back to the time I needed to adjust to my wife's death. Time does have a way to alleviate the heartbreak of death

We sat in silence for a moment. Mrs. Baxter seemed to regain her composure. "Can I ask you a question?" she said.

"Of course," I replied, knowing I did not have a clue what might be on her mind besides grief. Sometimes patient questions are elementary, but sometimes they become difficult and propose problematic scenarios that are more than complicated. The problems presented often threaten my ability to resolve them. Mrs. Baxter threw me for a loop.

"Does God choose when we die?" She was serious. It didn't sound like a spontaneous query that happened impulsively. No, I suspected she pondered this issue ever since the death of her husband a month ago. She had not, until now, reached the point of sharing her concern.

It had only been a few weeks since I buried Chester, and she was still in the throes of grief and missing him badly. "Chester was not ready. Why did God choose to take him now?" She expressed her anguish.

I felt wholly inadequate to respond with any sense of authority, but I took her question seriously. As a chaplain, I am regularly confronted with this concept, especially by those patients whose Christian faith takes priority. Death appears to be an elusive issue in the New Testament. Jesus talks about not fearing death. The fear of death prevents the person's freedom to live. When the fear of dying becomes all-consuming, little time and energy remain for living life entirely. Hence, the talk about death is merely a subterfuge to keep people focused on living fully. The serious Christian is never afraid to raise questions or express doubts, especially when it comes to a fixation upon death.

Some people, I have discovered, believe that there is a predestined day God has chosen for them to die. They don't think they have anything to do with it; fate determines it. Because God knows everything (I John 3:20), even the number of hairs on your head (Matt. 29:30), you can be sure that God knows exactly when, where, and how we will die. The Bible talks about a "book" in Psalm 139 that could be a reference to God's knowledge: *"All the days ordained for me were written in your book before one of them came to be." God knows absolutely everything about us* (Psalm 139:1-6). There is no secret action or thought that escapes His notice.

So…. does God know the day we are going to die? Do we have zero control over the time and date of our death?

The answer is mixed. Some say "yes," because God is omnipotent; God knows all and determines how all things will evolve and resolve. Some say "no." We do impact when we die; we can choose to jump off a bridge or drink poison, or manufacture a deadly car crash or other self-inflicted terminal circumstance. Any person can decide for himself if and when he wants to die and can accomplish that task in many ways; committing suicide by overdosing on pills or eating 100 Twinkies.

Rational thought was not what Mrs. Baxter wanted to hear. So, I kept my theology to myself for the time being, but it remained in my subconscious. I attempted to address Mrs. Baxter's concerns in more concrete terms. Her emotions were those of a grieving widow who was struggling hard to understand why her husband died; why God took him at this time when neither of them was prepared. I was struggling hard to offer some consolation and solace.

"God is not in the business of taking people's lives. God is not a murderer." I assured her. First of all, I wanted her to accept that from a Christian perspective, death is never in vain; it always has meaning.

"What meaning does death have," she asked? "I don't see that Chester's death was meaningful. What is meaningful about dying, unless it's a sacrifice for a cause, like Joan of Arc? Chester had more meaning when he was living." We both paused for a while as tears were beginning to well up in her eyes.

"Maybe thinking about it this way can be helpful," I stated. "A person is not ready to live fully unless he is ready to die." Then I remembered some spiritual thoughts from a past conversation that I shared with her. "There are many people who believe strongly that to live properly; we must live purposefully. Do you remember us talking about that before? Do you understand what they mean by that?"

"Chester lived a good life. I don't know that it had a great purpose other than to take care of his family, and he cared deeply about his country. He was a veteran who fought in world war two." she said

"He had a purpose in his life. Living his life accomplished that purpose," I said to her. "Purpose doesn't have to be complicated. Just living a complete life is purposeful."

I had with me a book of prayers and other sayings that I collected throughout my ministry that I could share with people at appropriate times. I remember reading to her what Martin Luther said. *"Even in the best of health, we should have death always before our eyes so that we will not expect to remain on this earth forever, but will have one foot in the air, so to speak and always given both the certainty of death and the uncertainty of when it will occur."*

I then told her, "I think God assures us that this separation is not permanent for believers like you and Chester. One day there will be a reuniting of the two of you in heaven, never to be separated again. For the Christian, this is what death is--it's setting sail, its breaking camp, it's being freed from this life so we can go home. "

I was unsure if the answer I offered Mrs. Baxter was sufficient or maybe a bit too esoteric, which clergy tend to be. Over time, however, she did grieve appropriately and began to move on with her new life. My feeling is that she was interested in gaining knowledge about the meaning of death; yes, but more interested in having someone with whom to share her feelings and allow her to vent.

Mrs. Baxter was not alone in her quest for meaning in death. There have been many patients who have raised the same or similar concerns. The question of whether there is a pre-determined date that God has chosen for people to die consumes these people.

As I stated previously, death and dying have a spiritual and religious dimension, at least from my perspective. I am supposed to think that way; people expect it. I am a chaplain, a spiritual counselor with hospice, a comforter of the terminally ill. As a chaplain, what I care about most is the patient's spiritual wellbeing, what provides mental comfort and security for that person right now, in the present.

I have confronted many folks who are serious about the concept that there is a pre-determined date God has chosen for people to die. Individuals have no choice; Fate strictly determines it. There is a sense of relief here for the believer.

On the other hand, some assert that dying involves choices. One can choose an optimal time and place. Strong feelings accompany one's choice, and people should be allowed to determine the location and time. The reasons for their choice vary from person to person and circumstance to circumstance.

For some hospice patients, suicide is one option. Patients ask to die when they have lost the ability to see a reason to live. Whether they take their own life or participate in some sort of assisted suicide, the motivation remains the same – "they don't want to live." Take, for example, Mrs. Karnes:

Mrs. Karnes' Story

Mrs. Karnes was a one hundred two-year-old lady who exudes grace and dignity and a heart as big as all outdoors. She lived in an assisted living facility. When I first encountered her as a hospice patient, I was astonished at her mental acuity and physical stamina. She carried on conversations in tandem with any group of people while comprehending the entire discussion. She demonstrated a vivid imagination and a specific recollection of both past and present memories. All this at one hundred two years of age.

However, it was not long afterward that I discovered that she was not the happy camper she appeared to be. She felt tormented by circumstances beyond her control.

"Tell me, chaplain, why does God let me live? I pray every morning that he takes me, but nothing happens."

"I don't think I understand," was my reply. Admitting ignorance sometimes is suitable for eliciting recent conversations.

She was sitting in a wheelchair. She seemed a bit tired and hesitated before she answered. When I first came into her room, I noticed that there was writing on the back of her wheelchair. "I have two great-great-grandchildren, 16 great-grandchildren,

22 grandchildren, and four children, all of them daughters. With that pedigree, I decided she could take whatever time she needed to respond to my query.

"Well…." she started slowly. "Well, I think one hundred two years is enough for any person to live, don't you? I feel blessed by God for the life he has given me all these years, but enough is enough. It's time for me to go, but God just doesn't want to let me. He doesn't want me to know when. You are a man of God. Tell me why God won't take me?"

My first reaction was that we were about to engage in some sort of deep theological conversation about the nature of God and why God does what God does. I was unprepared.

Then she surprised me. "This isn't rocket science," she added. "I just want to know why I am still alive when there is nothing else for me to do. I am ready, but it seems God isn't."

I gathered my thoughts. "Do you feel that God determines when a person dies?" I asked her.

"Yes, don't you?"

I changed the subject slightly. "Are you afraid to die?" I asked her

'No, not in the least. What's to fear?" Mrs. Karnes responded. "I just feel that I am ready and wonder how much longer I need to hang around and be of no use. My kids are ready for me to go. I am ready to go. I hope to go and be with my late husband. What's the purpose of my being here anymore?" She was beginning to cry, and I felt like I was the cause.

I was desperate to offer her words of comfort, but they did not come at that moment. We both sat for a while in silence. I had a hard time accepting that this one hundred two-year-old person could be so rational and contemplative. My experience with most people who might have reached her age was limited to observing them in a nursing home while they muttered incoherently to themselves and sat in the hallway and drooled. Mrs. Karnes was an enigma.

"Are you angry with God because he is not responding to your prayers?" I asked her.

"No, absolutely not," she assured me. I have great faith in God. Just look at my life. I am overwhelmingly grateful for the life I have. But now it's time to go, and I believe it will happen when God determines it. But I can't see any reason why God wants me to keep on living. I am not much use to anyone. I am not angry, just disappointed."

"Are you feeling depressed?" I asked. I was floundering, not knowing how to respond to her concerns. I never met anyone who wanted to end their life but was not depressed.

"I am not depressed. I feel blessed. I am grateful for all that life has given me. There is no depression here, only joy and satisfaction. But now, I have lived long enough and don't need to be around for people to have to take care of me. It's time for me to go."

At that moment, her oldest daughter arrived and barged into the room. She acknowledged that she was interrupting the visit from the chaplain. Immediately she inquired, "What are you two talking about?"

"Mom has some issues about her life," I responded. "No, I guess they are more about her death. She feels that she is ready to go and wants to die, but thinks that God is not helping her circumstance." I thought I needed to be forthcoming since patients' concerns, especially about suicide in any of its forms, demands an open conversation with family members.

"She is always talking about that," her daughter replied. There was a lull in the conversation as the daughter put away some of the clean clothes she had washed and placed them in her mother's closet.

"You know, mother, "she suddenly blurted out. "Our cousin John died just a year ago on this exact day. It was a sunny day, just like today. Today would be a good day for you to die."

I could not believe my ears. Mrs.Karnes's daughter suggested that today would be a good day for her mother to die. Mrs. Karnes just rolled her eyes and then stated, "She knows I am ready to go, and she just can't wait."

"Well, mother, if that is your wish, who am I to argue with you? Whatever makes you happy."

Each visit I made with Mrs. Karnes subsequentially included her request that it must be time for God to take her back. She never expressed any desperation or depression; consistently, she articulated her gratitude to God, reaffirmed her faith in Jesus, and demonstrated her positive perceptions about life. She continued her prayers for release from life. Time and time again, her daughter reaffirmed that same request but to this day, to no avail.

Thoughts one might have when recognizing that life is at an ending place can easily be those of premature death. That's understandable. However, such views are not always derived from feelings of desperation or despair, as is the case with more traditional suicide. Mrs. Karnes, who had no shame in saying she wanted to die and be with Jesus, felt it more as an honor. She felt proud to leave this life to be with God. Such thoughts have more to do with a clear understanding that life or death is more a decision of God than humans. I learned from Mrs. Karnes that suicide – assisted, merciful, or otherwise – is not just self-murder for the terminal patient; it is role–reversal with God. And so, for Mrs. Karnes, the great struggle is how to make it to God's appointed end, be it short or long, with joy, when your life is painful but faithful.

Mr. Taylor's Story

The Taylors lived in a trailer near the south end of Canyon Lake. The whole neighborhood consisted of trailers in various states of disrepair. Theirs was one of the least maintained. Junk was scattered all around outside - old car parts, a broken washing machine, empty bottles, plastic containers, and what looked like a year supply of McDonald boxes and wrappers.

My imagination consumed my thinking when in that neighborhood. I thought that maybe there was just one trailer, and that trailer got lonely and found a mate to move next door. These two copulated and gave birth to all the other trailers. How else can one explain why all the trailers look so much alike and remain in similar shapes. My imagination gets the best of me on occasion.

Mr. Taylor had a wife, three daughters, and a grandson all living together in the small home. Stuff was everywhere. A broken clothes dryer sat in a corner in the kitchen, taking up usable space. It was too heavy for the daughters to move outside and place next to the discarded washing machine. Cans and boxes of food -pancake mix, containers of cereal, laundry detergent, and dog food along with an assortment of utensils and kitchen gadgets, most of which appeared not to work, littered all the tabletop and cabinet space in the kitchen. A double bed sat in the middle of the living room. One had to intentionally walk around it to get anywhere else in the house.

Since Mr. Taylor was a hospice patient, we arranged for a hospital bed to be delivered. The only place it would fit was next to the double bed in the middle of the living area. Mr. Taylor wanted to be where he felt he was still part of the family and able to watch the large screen television that dominated one wall. Not much space remained in the living room except for a narrow path leading from the front door through the living room and into the kitchen area. The front door barely hung on since all the hinges were damaged and disheveled. I admired the family for honoring Mr. Taylor's request to be in the center of the living room at all cost to the rest of the family. They understood the importance of this to him.

The disease confined Mr. Taylor to that bed. He was not able to speak except for an occasional whisper. He was diagnosed with COPD, a particularly aggressive ailment that affected his lungs and halted his ability to breathe easily. Each breath was a struggle. This disease often sent him into fits of coughing that sounded like his insides were being blown out through his throat and mouth. He appeared almost comatose after one of these coughing fits that might last for at least a half-hour. The prognosis was that the disease would get progressively worse, and no treatment was available to reverse the momentum. In the early stages, oxygen relieves the symptoms, but during later stages, only pain medications offer respite. When asked if we could keep him comfortable during the late stages of the disease, not being a doctor, I hesitated to provide any guarantees. Not a sufficient answer for sure, but as a chaplain, that was not my area of expertise.

Today, Mr. Taylor could not speak or did not want to talk, at least not to me. His wife stood by my side as I introduced myself to him on that first visit. She attempted to interpret what he "wanted" when he couldn't say it himself. "He doesn't have any pain right now," she told me. It was hard to know if she knew that or was just guessing.

I smiled at Mr. Taylor, and he smiled back. I took that as an affirmation of what his wife just said; he didn't have any pain. "But sometimes he gets to coughing, and his face turns all red," she added. His facial expression indicated calmness and contentment at that moment, however. Reading facial expressions has become a visual sign I often count on to determine if a patient is presently in pain.

"I asked the usual first question. "What's most important to you right now, Mr. Taylor? I asked, already knowing that he didn't speak, but thought perhaps his wife might answer for him. His eyes caught my eyes, then shifted to his wife as if asking her to reply.

"I think I know what's important to him," his wife interjected. "He knows his grandson Clifford wants to get married, and he wants to be there."

"Can he get out of bed to get to the wedding, and when is it?" I asked her.

"I wanted to talk to you about that," she stated. "Can you marry people?"

"Yes," I responded. But I only people, not dogs or cats, only people." It was a reluctant attempt at a joke because I suspected what was coming next.

"Can you marry our grandson?' I expected that to be the question.

"Yes, I suppose so. When and where?"

"Here," she said. "And as soon as Clifford can get a license. Clifford wants his grandfather to be the ring bearer. Can we do it right here next to his bed?"

I looked around the room. The three very large Taylor daughters were sitting in the only chairs in the room, and his grandson was leaning on the television attached to the wall. All this, combined with the beds in the room, just about filled the space. Perhaps, I thought, if we both, Clifford and I, stood next to the bed while others watched from their chairs or the kitchen doorway, it was possible to pull this off. I took it as a challenge.

"I can do that," I sounded positive and emphatic, which I meant at the time, "But they will need to get a license, and I need to see it before we can do a ceremony. And I need to meet with Clifford and the girl he is marrying before we do this," I told them all

"We don't know how long Howard (Mr. Taylor) will be with us, so the sooner, the better. It's his last wish, the only thing that keeps him alive, to see them get married. He loves Clifford."

I asked Clifford what he thought about getting married.

"I'm gonna join the army, and I want to get married before I have to leave. Not sure when that will be for sure," he added,

"Who is your fiancé?

"Gracie," he said, "but she is not here. She has to be at work. But I can get here if you need to meet with her."

"If you want me to marry you, I need to know a little about the both of you and what your plans are to make sure you have thought this through." My query sounded a bit arrogant, but I have always felt strongly that I need to know there is some maturity to relationships, particularly the marriage relationship if I am the person who consummates that marriage. They also need to feel comfortable with me, although, at that moment, I felt that didn't matter too much to them.

"Let's set a time and date now. I will be back here again next week to visit with your grandfather. See if you can get Gracie here then, and we can make plans."

"Yes, sir," he said. "I will make sure Gracie is here."

About ten days went by before I set a time and date to visit again with Mr. Taylor. He was in the exact spot where I last left him, in bed by the front door. All the daughters were present; perhaps they never left. I don't think any of them worked. Clifford was there and introduced me to Gracie. We had the expected conversation, and we set a date and time for the wedding. Neither the groom nor Gracie had much to say and were more than compliant to let me plan the service.

The date for the wedding came sooner rather than later, and I arrived at the appointed time. Nobody was ready. Gracie retreated into the bathroom to fix her hair and apply her makeup. The daughters were busy in the kitchen preparing the different foods they had planned previously for the wedding. Clifford was outside doing some last-minute repairs to his car. Mrs. Taylor was busy moving furniture in the living area to make enough room for the few others they expected to be present. One guest showed for the wedding.

Mr. Taylor was in his bed. His hand was in a fist. I asked him to open his hand. He did, and the wedding ring was where it was supposed to be. He was ready to be the ring bearer and had a big smile on his face. No words, just a smile.

We all gathered together then, and I placed the bride and groom adjacent to Mr. Taylor's bed. I instructed Mr. Taylor to hand me the ring when I asked for it. Just as I was beginning the service, I heard Mr. Taylor snoring. He had fallen asleep, and as he did so, he relaxed his hand, and the ring fell onto the floor and slide under the bed. Clifford went down on his knees to retrieve it.

Just as I said, "And now I pronounce you and husband and wife," Mr. Taylor woke up. He had a surprised look on his face and examined his hands to discover he had no ring. His face turned despondent. His wife explained that he had fallen asleep, but the ring managed to get on Gracie's hand. Gracie bent toward the bed and kissed him. His smile returned immediately, and as a surprise to all of us, he erupted in a hardy laugh.

Less than a week later, Mr. Taylor expired. His wife, his three daughters, and Clifford, who had not yet joined the army, were devastated. They acknowledged that he was in a better place. They were convinced that he achieved his dying wish to be present at his grandson's wedding as an official ring bearer. They confided in me that they felt some grief but not overwhelmed because they felt confident that Mr. Taylor was content. Sometimes a hospice chaplain's responsibility is simply to be present regardless of what happens during that presence.

Chapter 14

Ariel's Story - A Visit to the Hospital Under Duress

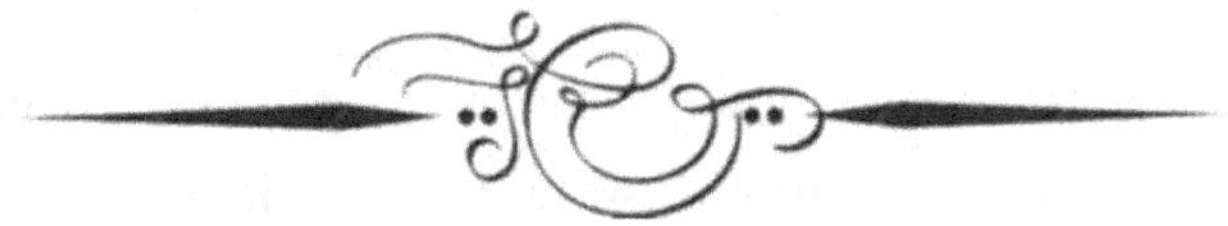

"A hospital bed is a parked taxi with the meter running".

- Groucho Marx

"Mom, how about we look for some other treatments? We got to keep working on finding a solution for your back pains." Both kids suggested this option at the same time. Ariel's response to suggestions she does something about her own health issues met with great reluctance on her part.

"When I need to see the doctor, I will let you know. In the meantime, don't keep harping on this," was her verbal response. Her physical reaction was much more forthcoming. She shook with pain. Sometimes the pain rendered her comatose. Her speech became slurred. Her appetite was non-existent. Her energy continued to wane rendering her energy closer and closer to zero. Still, she insisted all was well. Her recognition that she was in serious straights and needed therapy remained allusive; she just could not bring herself to admit that she had terminal cancer—very stubborn lady.

The one exception to her stoic responses was when her children elicited respnses. She could not say "no" to whatever they asked of her, regardless of its obscurity or insignificance. She was always a sucker for their appeals and gave in to their demands as a lover succumbs to roses on her birthday.

So….it was the kids who suggested Ariel seek further treatment, whatever was available to relieve her excruciating back pain. "Enough is enough," Kimberly told her. If you have cancer, and the symptoms suggest that it might be that, hospitalization seems like the only course for now."

We prepared ourselves for resistance. We expected some radical opposition from Ariel, but that didn't happen. She agreed. Something in her constitution had changed.

Going through the hospital emergency room seemed like the most efficient, easiest, and quickest means for getting her admitted. I performed the marriage for one of the emergency room doctors a while back, and he and I had become friendly. More importantly, Dr. Flanagan fully respected Ariel's talents, with whom he had worked closely when both were employed at the hospital. We counted on his willingness. We informed him on the phone that we wanted to bring Ariel to the emergency room. To facilitate the protocol required by the emergency room staff, he agreed to be present when we arrived.

"She is in serious pain," I informed the admitting nurse at the emergency room desk. Dr. Flannigan had already arrived and stood right behind her.

"She is one of my patients," he told the nurse. Immediately an attendant showed up with a gurney. We assisted Ariel onto a lying position on the gurney. She groaned while doing this, and I winced at her display of pain. They wheeled her into an examining room. I felt exceptionally fortunate to receive such a courteous and quick response in an emergency room. It was not how most people described their experiences here.

"It's her pain," I told the doctors who had come either out of curiosity or to assist. Ariel was well-liked by much of the hospital staff after her twenty-two years working there. It felt like it might be payback time. They gave her their attention.

"Can she get some relief from her back pain?" I asked whoever would listen. "I think her priority is relief from pain."

The doctors were pouring over her medical records that her doctors transferred to the emergency room. "Looks like she has tried all available pain meds," they told us after perusing her chart. One of the doctors suggested, "Maybe she might respond to methadone." It sounded like a suggestion more than a mandate.

Ariel was alert enough to hear and acknowledge the suggestion. "Do you want to try methadone?" I asked her.

"Yes." An emphatic "yes." No hesitation to think about it, just "yes." It was evident that she was prepared and anxious to submit to whatever therapy might provide some pain relief. She'd had enough pain to last a lifetime. Now she wanted it to stop, no more.

We waited for almost an hour for the medical pharmacy to formulate the methadone. Such a powerful pain reliever as methadone was highly restricted. Each patient and physician must comply with strict regulations. They soon informed her that she was eligible.

"Are you ready?" the doctor asked Ariel. She was still prone on the gurney but immediately sat up straight.

"Always a gracious person, Ariel answered, "Yes, please."

The doctor administered the medicine intravenously. I was not watching closely; however, it was all a blur at the time. I do recall sitting by her side, and after a few moments, her eyes began to close. She lay back on the gurney; we put a pillow under her head and covered her with a thin blanket, and soon she appeared to be asleep, deep sleep with heavy breathing. Her body relaxed.

"Her breathing is exceptionally heavy," I said to the doctor. "Is she having some sort of reaction to the drug?"

"No," he replied. "Ariel seems overly sensitive to the drug. It will cause her to sleep pretty soundly for a few hours, at least. We'll monitor her breathing."

I watched her face and noticed that all expressions of grimacing that I had grown used to disappeared. "She looks peaceful," Kimberly noticed. "Haven't seen her like that for so long."

"We need her to stay overnight," one of the doctors told us. I was not sure if he was suggesting or asking. He knew of Ariel's reluctance to be in a hospital as a patient and not as a nurse. "We want to observe her and take some tests."

We acquiesced despite knowing we might be the recipients of Ariel's wrath if she woke up at that moment and knew that we decided admittance without her consult. Perhaps, we were thinking; if she awoke and was already in the hospital bed, she might not object so rigorously. Her primary physician, Dr. Rue admitted her.

When Ariel arrived at her room, we found several hospital staff – nurses, aides, med technicians, dietary techs - already gathered there to greet her. She was well known and well-liked. They bent over backward to make sure she got premier consideration as a patient. Orders were left with the nurse that Ariel was to receive further pain medicine PRN (as needed). She rested comfortably for the first couple of hours, but the methadone began to wear off. Ariel became agitated. She even scolded the kids and me for "putting" her in the hospital. My feeling was that she knew she needed to be here. To relinquish, however, was to acknowledge that she needed medical help, which up to this day, she would not concede. I think I called her "stubborn" at that moment, but thankfully she did not hear me.

Ariel sat up in bed and told us, "Can you get the nurse to come and give me another dose?" Her request was another sign of her acquiescence; to want pain medication. I left the room, walked down the hall toward the nurse's station, and met the assigned nurse who was sitting and completing some computer data entry, so I assumed.

"Can you come and give Ariel, my wife, another dose of pain meds?" I asked her.

"Yes, I'll be there just as soon as I can," she replied.

I returned to the room. I trusted she meant what she said. Thirty minutes went by and no nurse. Ariel was getting anxious and antsy, not her usual composure. I thought we needed the meds now or even sooner. I returned to the nurse's station and found her still engrossed with the computer and eating a sandwich. I interrupted her.

"Excuse me," I said but got no acknowledgment. I tried again. "Excuse me. You said you would come to Ariel's room. We are still waiting. She needs her meds."

"I told you I would be there as soon as I can."

"But we need you now," I reiterated.

"Don't worry. I will be there shortly." She sounded annoyed.

I had no idea what "just as soon as possible" meant to her. I did know that dragging her feet or rebuffing us would not be tolerated. Once again, I returned to the room and waited. No nurse came.

The night supervisor who came on duty was the daughter of a friend of Ariel's with whom she worked at the hospital a few years back. I approached her, trying to remain composed as possible while seething underneath.

"The nurse assigned to Ariel is not being cooperative," I told her. "Ariel needs her pain meds and is not getting them. The nurse keeps putting it off and telling me she will be there as soon as possible, but it's been well over an hour and nothing yet." I could feel my blood pressure rising but did not lose my cool. Shortly, the head nurse appeared in Ariel's room with a vial of Ariel's medication, stuck it in her arm, and almost immediately, Ariel closed her eyes and fell back to sleep.

"I reassigned the other nurse," she told us. She would be Ariel's nurse from now on. "The first nurse was probably not a good fit for you," she continued, "so I am taking over." I thought that to be an understatement, to be sure.

"Thanks," I said. "I don't mean to belittle her. It's just that she was not responsive to us, as if our needs were not important."

For the duration of Ariel's visit to the hospital, the aides, the nurses, and others who attended to her could not have been more attentive and caring. I felt that most of the staff responded out of respect for one of their own who served in that hospital for twenty-two years.

Chapter 15

Resentments and Regrets

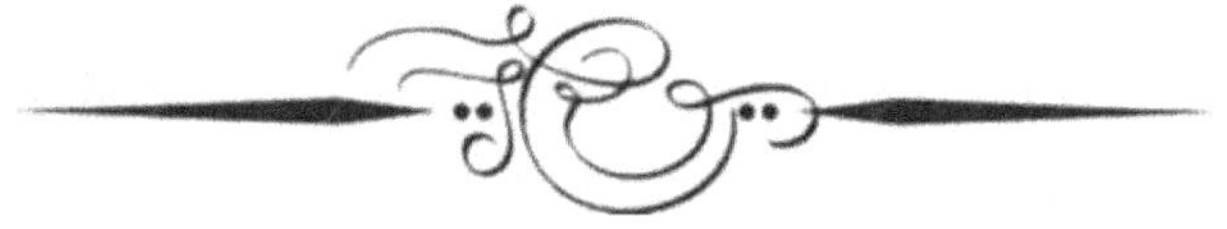

"Anger, resentment, and jealousy don't change the heart of others -- it only changes yours."

- Shannon Alder

Resentments and regrets, along with accompanying fears, creep up often and unsuspectedly for the dying person. To reflect on a life's experience just before death can recall episodes and occurrences that may have been buried deep within the soul for years. Almost obscure, these feelings come bursting forth with vibrant clarity, soon to overwhelm the patient with moods of anguish and torment. I have found these two "r's" (regrets, resentments) to be significantly detrimental and likely to trigger spiritual aches and pains in patients facing imminent death.

The movie *Rain Man (1988)* presents an excellent example of the consequences of holding resentments and regrets. At the beginning of the story, the younger son has a conversation with his girlfriend. He is recounting his feelings about when he wanted to take his father's antique Buick roadsters out for a ride. His father had explicitly denied that request and forbade him access to the car. One night, the son sneaks the vehicle out of the storage garage and proceeds to take it for a joy ride. He returns it safely. The father gets wind of the episode.

"I see you took the Buick out last night without my permission," the father says." He is visibly angry.

"Nothing happened to it," the son replies.

"That's not the point. I intentionally forbade you to drive that car, and you disobeyed me."

"I didn't hurt anything. The car just sits there. It needs to be driven. I did you a favor," the son also states with a tone of hostility in his voice.

"You knew you were not to drive the car, and you ignored my rules," There is more antagonism in the father's voice

"Well, I took it anyway," the son insists, "and I am not sorry."

Father and son move further and further into irrevocable mandates about who and what is right under the circumstances. Neither admits being wrong. They become estranged and unable to forgive for years.

Eventually, the father dies. The son is now lamenting forgiveness, that he never forgave his father nor asked him for forgiveness. He held the resentment tightly. He realizes it is too late for reconciliation with his father. He will carry his regret to his deathbed. It is a clear-cut case of placing principles above relationships; the concept that a person should not break a rule even if it means a relationship suffers.

Resentment is an issue I often encountered as I ministered to hospice patients. Indeed, resentment is not isolated to dying patients. It is generalized throughout the population, but it presents a particular problem with the terminally ill person.

Resentment occurs when a person repeatably replays feelings of hurt long after the initial circumstance that caused the harm. Recalling the emotion, we remember the feelings more than the facts. Since my patients tend to be among the elderly, I encountered people who carried resentments for years and years after the fact; people who could not let go of the feeling even after giving due consideration and analysis of the events for long periods. Patients adamantly held to their resentment despite friends, family, and professional advice to let go and forgive. They told me that "those who preach the benefits of forgiveness haven't walked in our shoes or felt what we feel."

But anger caused by resentment is not limited to the one person who precipitated the event. Anger is too intense an emotion to hang onto for long; anger eventually turns into indifference. Resentment goes global. Resentment can grow strong enough through the years to be directed not only at an individual but also transferred to other people. The person is not just angry at one person; instead, he becomes an angry person.

I have noticed that resentment rarely goes away on its own. It doesn't produce enough adrenalin that more potent forms of anger do. Exhaustion limits rage, but a person can stay resentful for years. When a disease becomes terminal, it comes out in full force. What's to lose, the patient reasons; I'm dying soon anyway, so might as well express the resentment.

Response to regret is similar to resentment. It only differs in kind rather than emotion. Regret appears to be associated with shame or guilt, shame for not accomplishing goals, and guilt for waiting too long. Regret tends to be a long-lasting emotion, but not one that has the mental torment of resentment. Most of my patients admitted to regrets, but only the anguished wanted to talk about their resentments.

Mr. Spahn's Story

Clayton Spahn, who joined our cadre of patients at hospice after suffering from severe heart failure, became an enigma to our entire staff. His conversations were confusing and sometimes paradoxical. What he told us about himself could be interpreted in a variety of ways. He had a myriad of opinions. He often communicated in opposites; life appeared diametric; something was one thing and at the same time another thing. For the duration of his stay with us, nobody figured him out, including his own family.

Clayton was a retired lineman with the telephone company. His job was climbing telephone poles, hocking up or unhooking the wires, and attaching the glass insulators used at the top of the poles.

When I was a kid, I had great admiration for pole climbers. I would watch in fascination as each man attached metal spikes to the side of his boots and then "walked" up the wooden pole almost as if he were a part squirrel. I wanted desperately to have a pair of these spikes for myself. I could climb just about any tree with ease, simply walk up along the trunk. To climb up trees like a cat seemed magical to me and would show me as the most admired boy in our neighborhood.

Clayton was equally proud of his position as a pole climber. He considered himself part of an elite group despite that pole climbing was a dying art, dying because telephone poles were no longer made of wood, but metal or concrete. Reaching the top of a telephone pole is now confined to riding in a bucket attached to a hoist's end on the back of a truck. Push the right buttons, and it brings you safely and directly to the top, where the worker can easily reach the wires.

"What was it like for you to be a linesman?" I asked him at our first meeting. Clayton was confined to his bed, unable to hold himself up by his legs. His face showed distress, even while resting in bed. He squinted his eyes until almost closed and held his lips tight together.

"Today Clayton sat up straight in bed, opened his eyes a bit, and said, "I liked it; liked it a lot."

I needed more conversation if I was to build a relationship with this man. I was interested in understanding what was most important to him; step one towards understanding his spiritual distresses.

"So, what was it about pole climbing that you enjoyed?" I asked him. "Was it dangerous?"

He hesitated a moment. He looked around the room, then out the window, and then back at me. "It was hard work, and I didn't like to work. But I did like to climb poles." His reply was my first hint at his paradoxical conversation. He didn't like work at the same time he did like work. He continued. "Even though I hated to work, I enjoyed being outside with my friends. I had good friends back in those days. We did the same kind of work. We got together once in a while, had a few beers, and talked bull shit." He was on a roll, and I encouraged him to continue.

"Sounds like fun on the job. Tell me more."

"We even had some competition. Who could climb fastest? We didn't speed at work, but when off work, the competition started. You know what I mean?"

We began our relationship limiting the discussion to mundane concerns – things he liked to do. What were his hobbies, how many years since he retired, and other superficial experiences? But as I began to engage him in what we refer to as "life review," I soon gained insight that all was not well spiritually with Clayton. By asking more probing questions, like what is most important to you right now and do you have any regrets, he began to reveal some conflicts with which he struggled. He told me about his two sons.

"They just don't like me."

"How long has this been going on?" I asked him

"I am not sure, but it's a long time."

Clayton had some dementia, and his memory about his sons' absence and other episodes remained fuzzy.

"Have you tried to make contact?" I asked innocently. I thought that there might be some rational explanation he could not remember. Maybe they lived too far away to visit frequently or had physical disabilities that prevented travel. "Can you call them on the phone?"

"They just don't come to visit me," he responded. "They just don't like me. It breaks my heart."

I stayed silent. I had no immediate response, only that I was glad that Clayton was willing to share his feelings with me. There was nothing specific to which I felt I could respond.

"It's hard knowing I don't have much time left, and now my sons don't want to come and see me. I don't understand. I don't know what went wrong."

"I'm sorry this has happened," I responded." You can't make them come if they chose not to. That has got to be their responsibility. Do you resent them?"

"Not really," he responded. "I just don't understand. I don't know what I did to deserve this?"

Having heard his response filled with remorse, and then observing his body language –the grimace on his face, the tone of his voice, the glower in his eyes - I suspected he was resentful even if he was unwilling to use that term.

The story Clayton told me was one-sided; I only heard his version. Clayton might be embellishing his story because of his hurt feelings. It might prove helpful if I could speak with the sons to learn if their perspective was different. They didn't respond to my invitation.

Instead, I had a conversation with his wife. I hoped she might cast light on the relationship. I needed a complete version of Clayton's story, so I could better understand the actual circumstances. I wanted to be prepared to intervene in his spiritual distress.

"That's right," Mrs. Spahn reiterated. "They have not been here in two years."

"Do they know Clayton's situation?" I asked her

I told them many times when I can get them on the phone. I have sent them emails and left messages. They know, but they don't respond."

"How did all this all get started? I mean, what caused this split?" I asked her.

"I don't know for sure. Since high school, they have been at odds with each other. Clayton was pretty strict with the rules. The boys had trouble with some of his rules. Clayton was never tolerant or understanding."

"Did things improve when they got older?" I asked her.

"When they were eighteen and nineteen, they both just moved out, and we've seen them only occasionally since then. Sometimes the boys came by when they thought Clayton was gone, but not if they knew he was here."

"So, what do you think about all this"?

Tears came to her eyes. She reached for the Kleenex box on the counter and pulled one out to pat her eyes. "It breaks my heart." She spoke quietly with intermittent sobs. "Of course, I miss them, but it's tough now with dad dying. I feel so bad for

Clayton. After all, they are still his sons, and seeing them before he dies is important to him. I feel like I let him down."

"It doesn't sound like you are the cause of the problem," I told her. "Sounds like it was Clayton's and the kids' stubbornness.

I realized what mattered was that reconciliation within the family was in danger of disintegrating. Clayton will go to his grave without recourse for reconciliation, and the kids will lament their guilt without the possibility of relief. They could avoid it if each side were willing to forego principles in favor of maintaining the relationship. Too often, I find families fragmented by stubbornness, claiming that they must stick by their hallowed principles even if it means family estrangement.

Clayton had firmly held ideologies to which he expected his children to observe without questioning. Unfortunately, his sons had minds of their own, as well as an inheritance of stubbornness from Dad. These were prescriptions for conflict. Neither Clayton nor the sons were willing to compromise their principles. Consequently, they remained estranged from each other. Reconciliation was not an option. They remained estranged for the remnants of Clayton's life.

Here is another clear example of how distressful and destructive resentments can be to a family. People become so entrenched in their holy principles that they maintain their refusal to budge even at this eleventh hour. Resentments will not die until ten minutes after we do.

After three weeks on our service, Mr. Spahn was declared active, a term meaning that death was on the doorstep. He had not eaten anything, no nourishment from food, nor was he consuming liquids. No one can stand that kind of torment for more than a few days.

Mrs. Spahn sat by his side day and night. She constantly wiped his lips with a small wet sponge. Breathing through your mouth, especially just before dying, causes the lips to be dry and irritable. She talked to him, reassuring him that she was present and that she would not leave him.

I knew the answer before I asked. "Have you heard anything from your sons?"

"No, nothing," she responded. Tears fell across her face as she spoke. She wiped them with a handkerchief she held in one hand while holding Clayton with her other hand.

"Tell me what you are thinking," I probed.

Slowly she spoke. "I can handle Clayton's passing," she said, "That's how it is supposed to be. But I can't handle the boys not being here. That's not how it's supposed to be."

Her real grief was not the impending death of her husband but rather her two sons' estrangement. She would adjust and adapt to his passing, but I am not sure she will recover from the feelings of devastation over the boys' absence. Dying comes inevitably and naturally. Family discord is far more devastating than death.

Marks story

Mark was a patient of mine suffering from heart failure. It is a standard hospice medical policy that patients be admitted for six months and then re-evaluated to determine if they remain eligible for hospice care. Medicare calls the shots here.

They decide who is qualified and who is not, depending upon the severity of their ailments. Mark fit that model well. Six months was just about right. He was preparing to pass on after six months. Some people have a sixth sense about a time to die. Mark was ready. He was in the hospital. I visited with him there.

I introduced myself as a hospice chaplain. Judging from his response, I thought him open to my presence and possible interference. I asked him point-blank, "What is most important to you right now? How do you want to spend the next six months?" This inquiry seemed abrupt, perhaps on first meeting a person but appropriate nonetheless.

The question of what is vital to the patient right now helps open conversation about the person's spiritual resources. Spirituality is almost always a measure of what each person finds significant to their lives, especially in the present.

"It's not easy to know where to start," Mark responded. "When I got sick, all I could think about was feeling better, recovering, and moving on. When I realized that was not going to happen, moving on meant to hospice. It became most important to know I would not be in pain, that you guys could control my suffering. Right now, I am not in pain, so I can begin to think about other things again."

"What other things?" I asked him. "What is most important now?" Having known him and his family for the past month, I felt like I knew a bit about how he thinks. So, I took a chance and asked him, "Any regrets."

There was silence for a while. Mark looked out the window. I wondered if I had touched a sore spot and maybe I should withdraw the question. His face, usually animated, turned solemn.

"Yeah, lots of regrets.

I reminded him about the nature of regrets and how they have to do with things undone, not something done.

Again, there was silence for a moment. I had second thoughts. Perhaps I treaded where I should have remained absent. Maybe I intruded on a subject that recalled too much pain for him. Nonetheless, I plunged ahead, aware of the risk. "What regrets are you thinking about?"

Slowly and purposefully, he began to lay out a litany of regrets. Each time he attempted to talk, I could see his brow furrow, and he would draw his lips tightly together against his teeth. He was in a zone that was painful for him.

"I have one brother, "he began. "We grew up the best of friends. We did everything together. We were less than two years apart. People thought we were twins. I went into the plumbing business with him after college and a recession. I was going to be a stockbroker, but it was not a good time. We began the plumbing business as a partnership, and for thirty years, we worked side by side, split all the profits equally."

"When he reached sixty- five, he just up and decided to leave the business. It came as a shock to me. He wanted half of what it was worth. I was not yet old enough to get social security, so I had to keep the business. I ended up paying him for his half of the business, which pretty much wiped out my entire savings."

"We parted ways, and he moved to a small town in New England and bought a house with his earnings. For the next three years, I never heard from him. I felt hurt that he left me in the lurch when he left the business. I didn't want to talk with him".

He continued with his story. "Two years ago, he died. I found out about it when his wife called one day. I was mad at him. But I knew someday we would get past those feelings and become close brothers again, but it never happened. Now it's too late. He died, and we have never forgiven each other. The regrets haunt me. It bothers me tremendously to this day." Tears began to flow again, and he reached for his hankerchief to dry his eyes.

"I understand what you are saying," I responded. "Maybe this is one of those times when only forgiveness can heal things."

"What do you mean?" he asked. "He's gone. I can't ask him for forgiveness now. I can't forgive him either because he is gone; he's not here."

"Yes, I understand. But forgiveness is a powerful tool for eliminating feelings of regret. I have been studying forgiveness for thirty years," I told him. "I still don't know why it works or how it works; I only know that it works." This idea was a mantra I had repeated with other patients as well. "Your brother doesn't need your forgiveness; that's past and can't be changed now. You are the one who needs forgiveness. You need to forgive yourself. The regrets are bottled up inside you and causing you great pain. Pain can be more than physical; it can be emotional or spiritual pain. You can get free of the pain of regrets by letting go of it and just forgiving yourself. Just let it go."

I felt compelled to offer an example of what I meant by "letting go" Probably a terrible example but the only one I could think of at the moment.

"You know, or maybe you don't know, that sometimes when a person gets drunk and feels nauseous, the best remedy is to throw up, get rid of what is inside you, let it go, and you suddenly feel a little better. Forgiveness works the same way. It allows you to rid yourself of what hurts, to let go of the pain of resentments." I urged him to try my remedy, and then I left.

I saw him again the following week.

"How are you doing with regrets?" I asked when first arriving. I was curious whether my suggested therapy might have worked or not.

"Still have some, but I am feeling more comfortable," he told me. I don't think he wanted to admit that I had been correct or helpful. "I shared what you said with my wife. We spent a couple of days together working on regrets for a whole bunch of things we both saved up."

I couldn't leave well enough alone and added, "Well, that's what hospice is all about – relieving pain."

Chapter 16

Ariel's Story – There is No Place Like Home Again.

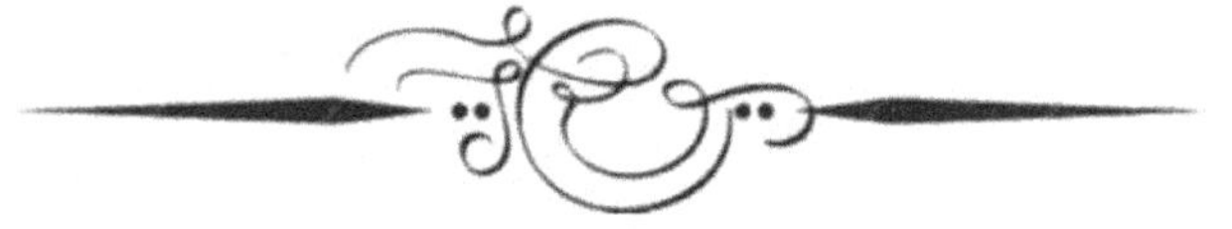

"It's a funny thing coming home. Nothing changes.

Everything looks the same, feels the same, even smells the same. You realize what's changed, is you."

- Eric Roth

Since Ariel was destined to be a hospital patient for however long, I decided to go home and get some essentials – pajamas, toiletries, Ariel's favorite cookies, and other "important" things; stuff without which she couldn't live. I returned with sleeping bags. Both my daughters determined they would not leave her side both day and night. No plans emerged yet as to how long she might be an in-patient. We would make decisions moment by moment depending on changing circumstances.

Early the next morning, we were startled by a cacophony of sounds outside her hospital room door. Word had spread among her friends and coworkers at Hope Hospice that we had admitted her to the hospital. In the hallways, about 10 – 12 hospice personnel had gathered. They were talking together. I went into the hallways to greet them.

After asking about her condition, they announced, "We want to keep watch. She is going to be one of our patients. We figured a way for her to be one of our patients without the lengthy paperwork. You don't have a problem with that, do you, Peter?" I knew better than to argue with a cache of assertive nurses.

The usual procedure with hospice was to assign one nurse to each patient. I knew this from Ariel's experience. It was beyond accepted practice to have a gaggle of hospice nurses assigned to one patient – Ariel. But seeing all these nurses gathered felt like a blessing I didn't deserve but was willing to accept. Their presence felt so comforting. It convinced me I need not worry about anything.

The feeling was short-lived, however. Presently Ariel's physician appeared and declared that he scheduled her for more tests. He prepared the tests to happen that morning. I don't remember what tests he planned, they happened quickly, and this same physician returned in the afternoon.

"I think we can conclude there is cancer in your system," he told us. We were not surprised, but hearing that word again brought on a certain sadness that slowly consumed each of us. The reality of the situation took our breaths away.

"I want to refer you to an oncologist," he further explained. "He will schedule you for a PET test to determine what kind of cancer is there before we think about treatment. It will take a few days to get the results back."

The idea of treatment had not yet sunk into my brain. I could only think about cancer as a death sentence. I could not bring myself to recognize that there might be a solution, a treatment that she could go through and come out smelling like a rose.

"What kind of treatments are you talking about?" I asked the doctor.

"Don't know," he responded. "That's what the oncologist will determine depending on what kind of cancer is in there."

The answer seemed too evasive; nothing I could lock onto that sounded like a real possibility. But despite my constant barrage of questions, evasiveness was all I got.

For the rest of that day, the hospice nurses remained present, not altogether, but one or two constantly at her side or outside the door. Ariel slept intermittently, depending on the frequency and amount of methadone administered. I was thankful for her peacefulness. The presence of the hospice nurses reinforced that peacefulness. It was not the peace of knowing that Ariel was to be healed and made well again, but rather the peace that comes knowing that we were not alone; we were comforted by the presence of others who truly cared.

Kimberly and Rebecca settled into the room. They had sleeping bags now, extra clothes, and toiletries. They were determined to stay for the duration. They refused to leave except to get something from the cafeteria. Ariel remained pain-free for the rest of that day. The amount of pain medication she received made her groggy, it slurred her speech, and she emerged in and out of consciousness. Her thoughts rambled, sometimes fairly lucid, other times incomprehensible.

The oncologist visited early the next morning. His conversation was less than inspiring. He wanted to do the PET test, yet her advanced cancer he already witnessed from previous tests convinced him she was probably already untreatable. Not the diagnosis we wanted the hear, but not entirely unsuspected either. Nonetheless, he requested that she come in for a PET test to pinpoint the exact nature, source, and whereabouts of the cancer. These efforts all sounded anti-climatical to me, and I registered my concerns.

"If you feel she is untreatable, why are we going through these tests? Besides, I am not sure we can get her to the lab you are suggesting for this PET test." He neither insisted nor acquiesced.

"Well, it's your choice," he said rather vaguely. He impressed me as if he didn't care one way or the other. My estimation of the doctor was an impulsive judgment and wholly unjustified, but rather an expression of my worn and fragile feelings.

The doctor excluded Ariell from these conversations. The medicines that brought her peacefulness also brought her sleepiness. Because of the oncologist's pessimistic diagnosis, combined with our understanding of Ariel's disdain for being hospitalized, it was an easy decision. We wanted to bring her home. Moreover, we knew hospice could provide care for her at home, if not better than in the hospital.

We recognized Ariel's terminal condition. We knew what Ariel would have wanted if we had consulted her. We decided for her. Tomorrow we would take her home.

Chapter 17

Families in Crisis

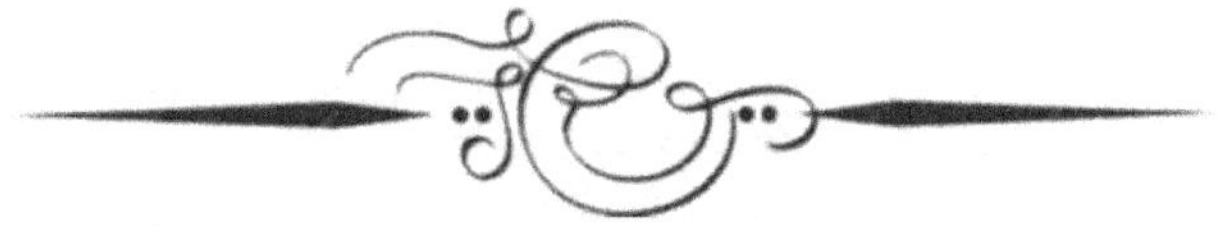

"In times of crisis, we must all decide again and again whom we love."

- Frank O'Hara

The sudden presence of terminal illness in a family can throw that family a curve for which they are unprepared. When they first learn that a family member faces a terminal diagnosis, folks will rally around that member. The family discusses resources and then makes plans. At this time, family unity is a priority, old grievances are pushed aside or put on hold. One or more of the family members, usually a spouse, takes the principal role of caretaker.

At this beginning stage, I have noticed that some upheavals are already pending that can disrupt the family caretaking. To acknowledge and live with the terminal disease can be stressful from the outset. Patients and families must make lifestyle changes. The home doesn't remain the same. Priorities shift to accommodate the terminally ill persons as well as the role of the caretaker. These changes are never welcomed and only reluctantly accepted.

The family members re-create their roles following the needs of the terminally ill person. Long-time issues, previously buried, can surface again under stress. Members find they reconstruct old family roles, such as planner, mediator, or problem-solver, which they feel they had shed many ions ago. They don't necessarily want to re-create these forgotten roles but feel forced to do so because of the new circumstances. Tensions can become particularly volatile when circumstances change significantly. The patient goes into remission or begins failing quickly.

Family members begin to feel guilty about the changing roles. They try to suppress these feelings, but they still underlie their emotions and eventually come streaming forth under stressful conditions. At this point, everyone's attentiveness is stretched, and their reserve of energy is dissipated. Nerves get strained, and patience wanes. As one caretaker suggested, "Managing the rest of my life has been so hard. Numbing exhaustion is a constant state for me – emotionally and physically. I need to keep going and do the right thing, but it's always in the midst of a crisis."

Life for the terminally ill might require a more extended period than first anticipated. This extension causes further stress. Both the terminally sick and the caretakers confront the need to "live with death" for a prolonged time. I pondered these thoughts as I share the following personal stories.

Mrs. Rheems Story

As a chaplain for Hospice, patients expected me to be present. "Being present" means having your focus, your attention, your thoughts and feelings all fixed on the task at hand." (CommuniCorp Group, 2012). The first encounter with a new patient has to be genuinely interpersonal. First impressions are like the first sentences of a good book; they must demand your immediate attention, or you move on to another book. I am sure that my relationships with certain patients that proved to be significant began at the first encounter. We connected immediately, and I was able to be "present" to them. Sometimes when we didn't click directly, we never recovered.

"I am not that religious" was her first response when I called to introduce myself to Mrs. Rheems as her hospice chaplain. "I have faith, and I go to church, but I don't spend a lot of time reflecting over religious stuff."

"I am not a preacher, "I assured her. "I Just want to know how you're feeling about being with hospice."

"Well, okay then, come on over." I was initially accepted. Now I had to prove my worth.

Mrs. Rheems was a new patient with a diagnosis of COPD. She had been assigned to me three days ago. Medicare mandates that new patients be visited the first time within a specific time frame. Today was the last day of that window. I was anxious to make contact.

Contacting patients for the first time was a struggle for me. I felt uneasy asking if I could come to their house. I felt as if I were intruding even though they requested hospice services. Because I thought I sounded apologetic when requesting a visit, I often called patients from the men's room. Most of the hospice staff was female, so I knew I had privacy in the bathroom. If the call sounded awkward, my coworkers could not hear my conversation.

"Good morning Mrs. Rheems. My name is Peter Olsen, I am a chaplain/counselor with Hope Hospice." which was how I introduced myself before she declared her religious preferences. I used the moniker of chaplain /counselor, emphasizing that the term sounded professional, easily accepted, and more closely associated with hospice. It wasn't, but it made me feel better. The word "chaplain" might be a turn-off. People often suspected that I was about to impose a sermon or try to evangelize them.

Having a chaplain as part of the hospice program was never obligatory; it was a choice. Hence, my reluctance when making the initial phone call was because of my fear of being rejected. I never entirely abandoned this anxiety and consequently spent many hours in the bathroom.

As noted above, Mrs. Rheems agreed that I could visit with her at her home the next morning. "But I have a pastor of my own and don't need religious counseling," she added.

I arrived on time. Her husband, Harry, met me at the door and ushered me into the kitchen area. Mrs. Rheems was seated at the kitchen table. A cup of coffee sat on the table in front of her. I could smell the aroma. Her hands grasped the cup and she took a sip.

"Would you like a cup?" Before I could answer, she said, "Harry, get the preacher man a cup of coffee. Be a dear."

The house appeared large. It overlooked a lake. I could see adjoining rooms from where I sat – the living room with lounge chairs and sofas, a den with a sizeable roll-down desk, the dining area with a huge oak table with six chairs surrounding it, and a swimming pool outside the back door. A cursory look around revealed they furnished the house with lots of antiques and oriental rugs. I surmised they were well off financially or had received a large inheritance.

"How do you feel?" I asked Mrs. Rheems. "Any aches or pains bothering you?" I have limited medical expertise, but the first part of all hospice assessments is to gauge the level of patient pain. Physical pain almost always has ramifications of spiritual or emotional distress, the bailiwick of the chaplain.

"No pain," she replied, "but lots of questions for you."

This declaration came as an unexpected request. Usually, the patient quietly sits while I drone on about the hospice services that will make life more tolerable. It usually takes more than a few visits before the patient opens up to personal concerns. Mrs. Rheems had given my visit some consideration before I even arrived. A book lay on the table.

"I have been reading some books about a man named Bonhoeffer," she told me. She pointed to the book on the table. I had a perfunctory understanding of Bonhoeffer, a German theologian who was part of the resistance movement against

Hitler during World War II. The Nazis's executed him for his opposition. I had not thought about Bonhoeffer since I was in graduate school many years previously.

"I don't like what he says about grace," she said. "The idea of grace has been on my mind for some time and since you're a clergy person, we need to talk about this." She reminded me quickly that Bonhoeffer's concept of cheap grace was hotly debated back in my seminary days, but I had not thought about this for decades.

"I got this bone to pick with Bonhoeffer," she interrupted my thought. "If what he says is true, then most of my Christian experience has been for naught."

She scared the hell out of me. I felt suddenly confronted and challenged by this lady I quickly categorized as a more astute thinking Christian than myself. When she discovers that I am a theological sham, a Christian slacker, a religious Charlton, she will reject me. I felt threatened by her brusqueness and intimidated by her awareness. These thoughts flashed quickly through my mind as I fidgeted in my chair and sipped the coffee her husband, Harry, prepared for me. I did not respond immediately. I felt numb.

Mrs. Rheems sat silently in her chair and stared at me as if waiting for my response. I managed to speak. "We can talk about that," I told her. "But can you tell me a little about yourself first?" It was a ploy to divert her, hoping that she might settle for some small talk about how God works in her life and what difference that has made as she lives out the rest of her limited life. But she was not to be swayed.

"You are trying to avoid these questions, aren't you?" was her immediate rejoinder.

She went on to inform me about her background. She was a retired teacher. She was active in her Presbyterian church, sang in the choir, and played her flute in the community band. At present, her congregation had an interim female pastor with whom she attempted dialogue about her theological questions, but it terminated without satisfaction.

"I have COPD," she reminded me. "I know I don't have much time left, and I can accept that. I think a lot about the shortness of time and the immensity of questions I have. I want to make some sense of my spiritual life now before it's too late. I am Christian, a believer, but I got doubts and questions. The religious stuff I can take or leave. It's the spiritual part that intrigues me. Bonhoeffer is one of the people I have read about, but I have to disagree with him if I read him right. If you don't mind my language, he pisses me off." She didn't mince her words or hide her feelings

She was just getting warmed up. Over the next few weeks, we continued to engage in theological conversation about all matters from resurrections to transubstantiation. However, she would not let go of her antagonism of Bonhoeffer and his concept of "cheap grace."

"He says we are all living under the illusion of God's grace, but in reality, we are cheapening that grace by the way we behave as Christians." I was amazed at her insight and grasp of theology. "I consider myself a decent Christian; I go to church regularly, pray, read the bible and try to emulate Jesus as best as I am able. I'm a good Presbyterian. For that, he says I am only exhibiting cheap grace. That pisses me off."

Not having a good retort, I encouraged her to say more. "Talk to me about what you mean. I am not sure I understand." A lame excuse on my part

She paused for a moment and then said. "I know I face death sooner or later, probably sooner. My faith has always meant the world to me. I can't imagine facing death without the strength of my faith. It assures me that I belong to God and won't be alone."

"And that is important to you, isn't it?" I asked.

"Yes, it is. Grace is God's gift to us, even if we don't ask for it. That's how I understand it anyway. But I did ask for it, but that's beside the point. What I hear Bonhoeffer saying is that it makes no difference. A lifetime commitment to Jesus always falls short. My belief in God is wasted effort because what grace I earn is given too easily, without deserving it. It sounds like he is saying, I don't deserve salvation. I am too selfish."

She paused for a moment and took a deep breath. I knew she had more to say, but her pause gave me a chance to interject a thought. "I am not sure you are reading Bonhoeffer right," I suggested. I feared that perhaps I was the one not well informed about Bonhoeffer.

She went on not acknowledging my contribution.

"Here," she said. "Let me read a quote about Bonhoeffer." *...cheap grace is the grace we bestow on ourselves. Cheap grace is the preaching of forgiveness without requiring repentance. ...Cheap grace is without cost...because it has been paid for everything and can be* *had for nothing*. Now that she had some ammunition, she lit into me like a tiger stalking a steak

She continued her tirade. "You mean to tell me that after all my years of faithful practice of the Christian ways, attending church, making donations, working at mission sites, and praying to Jesus as my savior that it was all for nothing? It's a fake faith? It's full of cheap grace? Isn't Bonhoeffer saying we're selfish if we expect our Christian faith to save us?"

She stopped, but I figured she was not finished, just exhausted. All this from a frail eighty-five-year-old lady whom the doctors diagnosed with a terminal illness. Such mental fervor without the physical stamina. I was beginning to realize that perhaps I was out of my league; I had met my match, and she relinquished me. `

Mrs. Rheems established that faith was of extreme importance to her, especially at this juncture of her life. She was not about to let some obscure theologian distract her, at least not without a battle. Her faith was her sole resource as she faced an uncertain future. But now, after reading Bonhoeffer, whom some well-meaning friend recommended to her, she felt her faith shattered and her spirit demolished. She thought she had nothing left, no resources to counter her fear about an impending conclusion to her life.

I felt I had sparse resources to offer her comfort and no sufficient apology that might relinquish her feelings of betrayal by Bonhoeffer; no way to fan the flames of her smoldering faith. As her chaplain, her spiritual counselor, I felt betrayed by my lack of understanding and compassion. I was not able to offer comfort to her from a faith perspective. I had nothing to suggest that would sufficiently alleviate her despair about "cheap grace."

We settled on a stalemate but agreed to tackle the subject again at future visits. I was encouraged that she agreed to have future visits. I felt that Mrs. Rheems stood by her contention that Bonhoeffer was a cad; that he diminished her faith by his instance on "cheap grace," which made her feel like a Charlton Christian, and she fell into a deep despondence. I made it my priority to find a way to restore her faith and provide her some spiritual comfort. I doubted myself. How could I be an agent of comfort, when I failed to reassure her that her faith was "blessed assurance" and sufficient to carry her beyond skepticism.

One week after our last conversation, during which I was less than convincing in alleviating her doubts, Mrs. Rheems decided to pursue aggressive treatment for her COPD. When this occurs, the patient is no longer eligible for hospice services. Her last words to me before she hung up the phone after saying goodbye were, "I'll be back. You haven't heard the last of this. We will continue this conversation, mark my words."

She did not return, at least not right away. My reaction to our relationship remained in limbo. Her trust in me, whereby she felt comfortable sharing intimate feelings and thoughts, gave me gratification. Still, my ability to resolve her concerns and doubts about her faith left me feeling inadequate. I was both challenged and enriched by her confrontation.

Mr. Rheems Story

When I looked at the morning R and A report (referral and admission), I immediately noticed one of the new patients was Harry Rheems. I said to myself because no one else was listening, "This must be Mrs. Rheem's husband. I forget his name was Harry." Mrs. Rheems was one of my favorite patients from almost one-year past. She never died; she just got better and left hospice care. I have had no subsequent contact with her or the family since. When she was on hospice, Harry was her primary caretaker, but I hardly ever saw him upon my visits. At that time, I thought him not to be deferential toward me. He never entered into the conversations I had with his wife. Instead, he stayed in another room and only appeared to say goodbye.

Mrs. Rheems, as I remembered her, was a slight lady somewhere in her early eighties. She had a sharp mind, inquisitive about many subjects. She sang in her church choir and played the flute in the church band. Her church was the center of her intellectual life as well as her social life.

Despite looking a lot frailer than average, she excelled at holding her own in a conversation. Never afraid to voice her opinion. She did not fear engaging in conversation with someone she held in great esteem or had academic degrees that surpassed her own. When engaged in conversation about theological and religious circumstances, her questioning showed a high degree of knowledge far beyond her estimation of being "just a housewife." I often felt that she purposefully underestimated her ability to gain the upper hand of an unsuspecting person with whom she was conversing like the professional pool shark who intentionally uses the ploy of not knowing which end of the pool cue to use to lure the inspecting gamer into submission.

I instantly recalled the opinions she shared regarding theological queries, precisely, issues focused on Dietrich Bonhoeffer's work. She consumed hours investigating and evaluating Bonhoeffer's theory of "cheap grace," a concept she could never assimilate.

"I would like to be the chaplain for Mr. Rheems," I told the supervising nurse who was in charge of assigning clinical staff. "His wife was one of my patients last year until she left hospice. We were pretty close," I added. Adding "close," I suggested that I would be the best fit for the family since I had a history with them. That counts for much in the chaplain/patient relationship in hospice.

"She already requested you," the nurse told me. "Get in touch as soon as you can. He came on service three days ago, and we let it slip because Alva (the admitting nurse) was out. Got just a few days to do the initial eval." She added.

I went into the bathroom and took my cell phone with me. I called Mrs. Rheem's home. The bathroom provided me privacy. I had no separate office, only an alcove adjacent to other staff in nearby alcoves. I didn't want others to overhear my conversations.

"Good morning Mrs. Rheems. It's Peter Olsen, the chaplain at Hope Hospice. I don't know if you remember me, but hospice asked me to be the chaplain for Mr. Rheems."

"Of course, I remember you, Peter. Didn't they tell you that I specifically asked for you?"

"I appreciate your confidence. I remember the talks you and I had last year. I hope all is well with you."

"I still wish I was on hospice, but I was not eligible anymore after my surgery. And, yes, I remember our talks together."

"Can I set a time to come by to visit with you folks? I need to see Mr. Rheems as soon as possible if that is convenient for you.

"Let me check with Harry," she said. "Things are different this time. I am not the sick one. Harry is, and all this has been upsetting for the whole family." She turned away from the phone, and I could hear her addressing Harry. "Harry, it's Peter, the hospice chaplain. He wants to know if he can come and visit."

"Who?"

"Peter, you remember the chaplain from hospice that used to come and visit with me."

"No, I don't" was Harry's response.

Mrs. Rheems came back to the phone. "Harry is having a lot of trouble remembering things," she told me. "At times, he becomes uncooperative, and that concerns me, but if you can come by soon, maybe you can help calm him down and me too. You do understand that at any time, he might fall asleep, and he is difficult and agitated when we wake him up."

I told her I understood. I would be there in the morning. In the meantime, I read the admitting nurse's report. Harry was diagnosed with Lewy Bodies, a type of progressive dementia that eventually leads to a loss of attentiveness, possible hallucinations, and likely Parkinson's disease symptoms. On top of that, his heart was failing. The nurse indicated that he responded erratically to her questions, not always making sense but didn't complain of any severe pain. She noted that his wife, Mrs. Rheems, was upset and distraught, more than the usual spouse might be when assuming the care for her husband. I noted this observation.

I arrived at 10:00 the next morning. Mrs. Rheems greeted me at the door. I said, "Hi, good to see you again." She stared at me for a moment, and before I could say another word, she reached forward and hugged me. As I followed her into the house, she reminded me, "I have missed our conversations. I remember them well. Even though we rarely agreed, the talks were meaningful. You helped me more than I think you know to come to grips with my spiritual life. Things have changed here. Now it is Harry who is the sick one, and I am his caretaker. When you were here before, things were reversed. I was ill, and Harry took care of me. He was in good health then, and things changed so quickly.

"It sounds like it has been challenging for you to reverse roles with Harry," I told her.

We sat at her kitchen table for a few moments as she seemed anxious to talk." Yes, very difficult," she said. "I always thought Harry was the healthy one, and I would go long before him. He felt that way also until this happened. We had long conversations back then about how Harry would live his life alone after I died. Now, when he is lucid, we talk about the same things, only the roles are different. I am not handling this well. "Tears began to well up in her eyes.

"Does he know about me? Does he know I am here?"

"I don't think he remembers," she responded. He doesn't always have clear thinking. He gets confused quickly, and sometimes he becomes agitated, which frightens me."

I interrupted her. "What do you think is most important to Harry right now?" I had to get that question in somewhere.

"I don't know for sure. Some days he is lucid, and some days I don't know what he is saying. He talks in circles. The girls (their daughters) try to keep him calm, but it isn't easy. I am hoping you can help calm him down; give him some assurance that he is okay. I am sure he is aware that he is not well."

At first, I felt overwhelmed by Mrs. Rheem's request. It sounded like a tall order. I might not be able to accomplish that. Mainly because of our history, I did not want to disappoint Mrs. Rheems.

"Let me go and visit with Harry," I told her. "We can talk after that."

Harry had just awakened from a morning nap. He appeared groggy and confused. With some persistence on my part, he eventually stated he remembered me, but that might have been a diversion to cease my persistent and annoying questions. I am sure that has happened with other patients. What responses I got indicated that he was neither in severe physical pain nor emotional stress. I turned my attention back to Mrs. Rheem, who was waiting in the living room.

She had no hesitation in describing her anguish. "I feel so guilty," she exclaimed. And then she posed the penultimate question. Am I less a Christian because I don't want to care for him myself? I have become one of those Christians that Bonhoeffer refers to as relying on *"cheap grace"* that I railed against before? I feel like a Christian hypocrite. I don't want to keep my end of the Christian bargain. I am living cheap grace.

"Hold on a second," I suggested. I hoped that Mrs. Rheems would not take umbrage with my abrupt comment. I wanted to redirect the conversation away from a discourse of religious doctrines and refocus on her particular emotional struggles. "It sounds like you have great stress, caught between keeping him at home or placing him in a facility."

"Yes, that has crossed my mind, and I don't like thinking about that. The girls have asked me about that as well. It just feels so wrong to take him away from his home, our home. I feel like I am deserting him."

We were both silent for a few moments. Again, tears welled up in Mrs. Rheem's eyes. "There is a lot that goes into making that kind of decision," I suggested to her. "If he stays here, it will mean a lot of hard work for you and will probably exhaust you. I think you know from talking with other people that it means long hours and a requirement that you give up much of your normal life. Some people come to resent that and then resent the people they have to take care of."

I gave her some time to cogitate on that. I continued. "That can hurt the relationship you two have; you start to resent Harry for upsetting your life so drastically. Think about the alternative. If he is cared for in a facility that relieves you of the exhausting work, no resentment about that, and when you visit, you can spend quality time with him. Either way is a crapshoot."

"But what about the guilt?" she asked. "I am sure that guilt will follow me."

"Well, there may not be any full-proof resolution for feeling guilt. Just because someone says you should not feel guilty doesn't mean it magically goes away. The only thing I can suggest is that you forgive yourself for making what you feel is the best decision and get on with your life. Once you decide, don't try to second guess it by saying you should have done something different. Stay with that decision." I left her to contemplate my suggestions and counsel.

About three days later, when I next called her, she informed me that she had already registered Harry in the Eden Home Assisted living facility. She was talking to me on her phone from there at that moment."

"Can you come up here today?" she requested.

"Be there in about half-hour. How's Harry doing?"

"Not well today. He's confused and angry," she replied.

"We'll talk about it when I get there."

The Eden Assisted Living facility was a relatively recent addition to a nursing home complex that has been in the community for many years. The home earned an excellent reputation as a caring facility throughout its tenure in the community; it possessed excellent nursing care, a good patient/staff ratio, and well-maintained quarters. None of these places come cheaply, however. Room, board, and medical/nursing care are quite expensive, usually beyond most families' financial capacity without long-term insurance or not poor enough to qualify for Medicaid. The Rheems met neither of these criteria; they were too poor to pay full fare and too rich to receive Medicaid assistance.

I arrived about an hour later and met Mrs. Rheems just outside the door to Harry's room. After a brief greeting and response to "how you doing," she immediately said, "This place is going to take every penny we have left."

"It's hard to know if you made the right decision, but you made a decision, and it sounds like you did it for both of you," I responded. Mrs. Rheems then added a concern.

"Karen (one of her daughters) is distressed. She thinks dad should be at home, that it is his wish to be left there and that I should honor his wishes. She is pissed. She just left."

"What about your other daughters (she had two more)?"

"They're alright with the decision. They said they could visit Dad here just as easily as at home. It's closer to where they live and work. I don't know what to do? Or know what's right?" She started to cry, and I put my arms around her.

"This was not supposed to be this way," she told me. "I was supposed to be here, not Harry, and now I feel guilty and confused. Even my kids think I am horrible, at least Karen does."

"I wish I had an answer for you," I told her. "You had to decide, and it sounds like you gave the decision good consideration. Trust your instincts a bit. You are acting out of love and care, and you don't need to diminish that feeling no matter what other people think."

Mrs. Rheems stopped crying and wiped her eyes. She then looked up at me and said, "Cheap grace, remember when we talked about that. That's what I am feeling now, like I committed cheap grace."

Over the next few days, I was able to gather the entire family together. They shared feelings about the move, but more than that, they shared feelings about Harry, their father. The expressions of mutual consideration about his welfare and how they felt they were responding to his needs allowed them to reconcile and settle in on the best solution – Harry needed the extra care that Eden Home could provide.

Mr. Reinhardt's Story

Mr. Reinhardt was a Texas rancher (not to be confused with a farmer). He owned and worked about twenty-five acres of bottomland covered with sage bush, low juniper, and prickly pine native to the area. In Texas, having steers, not cows, distinguishes a rancher from a farmer. In this part of Texas, many of the ranchers were descendants of the original old German settlers. They inherited the land and the cultural habits and customs of being extremely independent and quite naturally stubborn. I knew him because, in my previous life as a pastoral minister, his wife was once my church secretary. Both of them were church members. Now Mr. Reinhardt became a patient of hospice, and Hope Hospice assigned me as his chaplain.

One day, his hospice nurse contacted me and told me that she was a bit frightened by their last conversation together. "He told me he was thinking about suicide. I know he has a gun in the house. He says he would like to go to bed some night real soon and just not wake up in the morning. That makes me think he is willing to do that, and he has a gun or enough meds to make that possible. Can you and Sonia (the hospice social worker) intervene here?"

I agreed and made contact with Sonia to schedule a visit with me. I did not know, nor did his nurse know, whether his wife was aware of his tendencies. I agreed to contact her to let her know of our concern and to schedule a family conference.

"He's always talking like that," she told me when I called his wife. "He's been threatening to kill himself for years. Whenever things don't go the way he wants them to, he always says he will go out to the barn and shoot himself. I used to worry, but after so many times, you get used to it. His grandpappy was just like that as well and didn't die until he was ninety-six."

I reminded her that if our staff suspects a possible suicide, even if unlikely, we are mandated to address it. If we judge it not seriously, fine, but we cannot ignore it. Hence, we need to confront Mr. Reinhardt and have a conversation. His wife eventually agreed. I set a time and date for the meeting.

"So, what is this meeting all about?" was Mr. Reinhardt's first response as he sat down at the table. He had a puzzled look on his face, and his eyes were glancing around looking at each of us. He eventually settled on his wife. "Did you ask for this?" he addressed his wife directly.

Mr. Reinhardt is in his middle eighties. He has been a farmer and rancher all his married life. He admits to not knowing much about life other than ranching but does insist that he is a damn good "cattle caretaker," as he likes to say. Right now, he is greatly hampered by being unable to walk by himself. He uses a wheelchair and complains about pain in his legs constantly, both of which are symptomatic of his terminal heart disease

He continues to consider himself self-sufficient despite little that he can do about the ranch - he can't feed the cattle, can't cut the hay, can't plant the rye. Nonetheless, he insisted there was no reason why he could not get on his tractor. "Been driving that tractor for thirty years. Don't need to stop now," he maintained in defiance of his family's ban on dangerous activity. "I will drive that tractor till God himself pulls me off."

One day he convinced his son and wife he was fully capable of controlling the tractor. Because of his stubbornness, they gave in and helped situate him in the driver's seat where he could reach all the controls. He started the tractor and drove off toward the barn.

However, this day, because his legs were partially immobile, his left leg got caught against the throttle pedal. He could not untangle his leg to release the gear which he had set in forward. Consequently, the tractor lurched forward until it met the barn's unmovable force where it came to a halt, and the motor stalled.

Fortunately, Mr. Reinhardt was not seriously injured. His pride took a beating as he agreed that tractor driving was no longer an option. Today, he was back in his wheelchair as he came to the table. We continued the conversation we had begun.

Addressing his wife, he again asked, "Did you ask for this meeting?

"She knows about it," I responded, "but we, Sonia and I, asked for it and thought she needed to be present." I continued, "Last week, you shared with the nurse that you wanted to end your life, and when we hear something like that, we have to talk with you about this. Do you understand why we need to talk with you?"

He looked sheepish, like a child who got caught in a lie. He squirmed in his chair, looking around the room but not directly at any one of us. We waited for a response.

"Yea, so?" he responded with his German accent. His tone sounded like a question. He fell silent, but not for long. "Why should I go on living? My heart doest's work right, and I'm going to die soon anyway. I can't get on the tractor; can't feed the cows. I can hardly walk and have to use a wheelchair. What kind of life is that anyway?"

" So that means you want to take your life now?" I asked him.

"All of you will be better off if I die. I am useless now and a burden to Marilyn (his wife). It would be best for all if I died now." He sounded angrier but not apologetic

Marilyn protested. "You are not a burden, and I don't want you to die."

There was some back-and-forth conversation about whether he/she felt he was a burden. I interjected. "What if

Marilyn tells you that she takes care of you because she wants to, not because she has to?"

He fell silent at that question. I presumed he was thinking.

"I am a burden to the whole family. I can't go to the bathroom by myself. I can't take care of the cows. Marilyn has to feed them in the heat of the summer." His voice got louder and more distressed. "I can't stand having to rely on other people. If I can't do things the way I have always done them, I don't want to do them at all. I'd rather be DEAD." He emphasized being dead.

"Can I tell you about my father?" I asked him. It's not the best therapy to talk with patients about your personal life, but I felt the story might make an impact at this point. I was desperate.

"My dad had prostate cancer. It affected his legs mostly, hard for him to walk or stand for any length of time. When he visited with us, I always encouraged him to come out to the garden and check out my tomato plants. Tomatoes were his specialty in his garden.

I showed him how I pinched off the sucker shoots just like he had taught me because it allowed the main shoots to grow better. 'Can you help me pick off the suckers' I asked him?"

Suddenly he turned and walked back into the house. His abrupt departure concerned me, so I followed him. "What's the matter?" I asked him.

"Peter, I can't bend down anymore to reach the tomato plants. If I cannot do that the way I always did it, I don't want to do it at all."

"That made me think about coping strategies. What if I get a small stool, and you can sit down to pinch off the shoots?" I got a small stool. Reluctantly he tried it. After a bit of adjustment, he found it worked for him, not like it always did but like it needed to do now. He learned to cope, not give up."

I finished my story. No one responded with any comments. I could not tell if it impressed Mr. Reinhardt or bored him. The suspense was too great. Sonia interrupted the silence.

"Have you thought about how your death would affect your family? If you were to die, let's say tomorrow when you could be living another few months or longer, how would it make them feel to lose you early?"

His wife, Marilyn, jumped into the conversation. "Ever since you got sick and the doctor said it was terminal, I have lived knowing I would lose you eventually. But you are still around, and some days you are doing fairly well, with no pain and able to do some things you like. I enjoy every minute of that and want it to continue as long as you are able. If you kill yourself now, I won't have that time with you."

Her response motivated Sonia. "Won't it be selfish for you to take your own life now? You have said that your family is the most important thing in your life. They want you to be around for a while; enjoy your company. If you kill yourself, you are depriving them of what little joy they might have. Killing yourself, that's telling them they are not important to you."

I felt that Sonia might have touched a nerve with him but perhaps not. After a few moments of contemplation, he said,

"You won't miss me. You will be a lot happier when you don't have to take care of me anymore. I am nothing but a burden and better off dead. I got no future, only more pain."

Because the conversation was becoming extremely tense and I sensed that Mr. Reinhardt was feeling buttonholed to reconsider his feelings about suicide, I suggested that we back away for a while, take a breather, and have a cookie. Mrs. Reinhardt had placed a plate full of molasses cookies on the table earlier, but we had not partaken as of yet. I didn't feel that Mr. Reinhardt was ready to make concessions, nor had he been sufficiently convinced that suicide was not his best option. I did think that we had opened possibilities worthy of his consideration, and if given some ample time to reflect, he might not be so hasty to end his life.

Bottom line – we confronted the circumstances as best as we were able. How Mr. Reinhardt would react remained his personal decision. Only time would determine the outcome. We finished the cookies of cookies while conversing about the hardships of ranching and the recent weather extremes.

Upon reflecting, I thought Mr. Reinhardt exhibited some of the same characteristics that others have regarding suicide at the end of life. Each person concludes that life must end, but for various reasons. For some, it is a quest for a peaceful solution to a life lived too long; long enough that being anxious to pass on is a spiritual quest of completing what is essential to that person – being called home by God.

For others, the consequences may be similar to end life, but the circumstance reflects a different perspective. If death is the consequence of the terminal sickness, let's get it over with now.

We do not need to prolong suffering. There are deep feelings of becoming a burden to loved ones, and death releases the burdensomeness.

Brian's Story

Resentment is when you feel someone has wronged you. It has no physical presence. Instead, it comes barreling down on you with a strong emotion that feels heavy for a long time. It can arise spontaneously when least expected. Sometimes a particular event will trigger resentment in the terminally ill patient causing great havoc among family members.

Take for example, Brian, a patient under hospice care. His wife Sherri and he took time to explain how they got into this fix which eventually brought him to hospice. In his early fifties, Brian was now living in a mobile home in Texas after a long time in Alaska. He spoke fondly of his days spent in the "great outdoors of the north." His wife Sheri lived with him, and his daughter rarely visited due to tensions between her and Sheri.

Brian was diagnosed with heart failure and given a terminal date of six months. Six months is an arbitrary number assigned by Medicare as required for hospice eligibility. Not all patients make it to the sixth month, and some remain long afterward and become recertified for another six months.

When I first met him, he was comparatively active for a person with heart disease. His home was near the edge of some woods. He and his wife haphazardly decorated the inside with an assortment of couches, stuffed chairs, side tables, and a large screen television mounted on one wall directly in front of the bed Brian was occupying in the living room. Having the bed in the living room was a recent addition. Brian had decided that since he had to "rest" so much due to his condition, he did not want to be isolated in the bedroom. Besides, the large screen allowed him virtual access to Alaska wildlife films.

"I was doing fine until the accident," he told me when I probed about his circumstances.

"What accident?" I asked in response. Brian had a habit of taking time between his sentences and did not always reply immediately to questions posed to him.

"An accident," I repeated while waiting for Brian to respond. "That sounds horrible. Can you tell me what happened?"

Brian impressed me from the first time I met him as somewhat introspective, a bit allusive in his conversation, and modest. Taking his time to answer questions, I interpreted his contemplative interlude as a time for him to consider the request before responding. When he answered, he often attempted to redirect the subject which I construed as his reluctance to deal with personal feelings. Besides, he indicated he felt uncomfortable whenever his wife offered words of praise or support. He prepared me for hesitations if I asked him to share his feelings. But he acquiesced. He told me his story.

"Sherri and I were on route 316 heading into town one morning (Brian paused between sentences as if contemplating his next thought before continuing conversation). I can't exactly remember what happened…I think I was reaching for my phone which dropped into my lap or onto the floor…Suddenly Sherri yells at me loudly *GET BACK ON THE ROAD BRIAN*…It so startled me that I looked up and saw we were heading off the road….and I tried to correct it but overcorrected, and we slammed into a tree by the side of the road."

Sherri interrupted Brian. It was easy to interrupt him because he took so long to finish each sentence. Sherri's body language clearly showed annoyance. She was anxious for Brian to complete his explanation.

"It was horrible," she stated. She talked extremely fast. "The whole front of the car collapsed. The steering wheel ended up between us. We didn't pass out or anything like that, but we were stuck in the car and couldn't get out." She let Brian continue to describe the accident

So, Brian continued. "Some passersby stopped and tried to help us but could not budge the car door…. They called 911… and about twenty minutes later they arrived along with a wrecker truck…. (Brian pauses). I think I was unconscious most of that time. I don't remember feeling any pain…..But it turned out that I had broken one of my legs and lots of internal damage."

Sherri went into the other room and brought back a picture the EMS people took of the car. It showed the front end completely demolished, mangled as if crushed by a large rock.

"That you escaped without being killed must have been a miracle," I stated. The picture made me gag. Both Sherri and Brian appeared unimpressed by my spiritual explanation.

"I was in the hospital for a few days," Brian said. "They wanted to take a few tests…; they always want to take tests. They set my brace for my leg… That's when the worst part came….They said I had a heart condition that wasn't good….They said they couldn't do reconstructive surgery on my leg because my heart's weakness would kill me during the operation….So I am really in the hospital because of my heart, not the accident."

"That's quite a turn of events," I said. "Sounds like you weren't expecting that."

"Yeah, really screwed up my life."

I had pegged Brian as wanting to be independent and stubborn person. What he told me next verified my hunches.

"I got pissed," he said. "Everything was fine, I thought…..I could do what I wanted to do, like go back to Alaska hunting again or shoot my guns at the range or fishing…I was planning to go back to Alaska, maybe even move there, but that's all just a dream now. A nightmare…. Because they said something was wrong with my heart, I got to be on hospice now and can't do nothing."

"So, who are you pissed at?" I asked him. "You mad at God, like it isn't fair God. Why me?"

"No, I don't think much about that stuff. Religion is not a big part of my life. I can't blame stuff on that…..I just get really upset when I can't take care of myself….Sherri has to do most of the stuff around the house now….She has to take care of me, and I don't like being taken care of….I get pissed at Sherri cause she has to take care of me, and I don't want that. It makes me feel shitty about myself."

I could sense his frustration. When his wife had to meet his needs, take care of him, do something he usually could do himself, he reacted in anger. Brian would lash out at Sherri.

"I just want to help you," Sherri piped in.

"It's not helping," Brian yelled back. "You know how I feel about having you treat me like a little child." His attitude expressed great annoyance as he raised his voice to a feverish pitch.

Sherri would rage back at him. "I'm trying to be of help to you." Like Brian, she verged on yelling. "I am your wife, and that's what wives do; they help their husbands. But you don't respect that, and you treat me like shit." And almost immediately, she added with a loud, harsh voice on the verge of tears, "Sometimes I wish you would go ahead and die. That would stop your abuse of me."

Brian paused for a moment and then said, "Just stop babying me. I would rather be dead than to have you always telling me what I should do; what I ought to be doing…..I'm tired of you always being in my face." Both Sherri and Brian had grimaces on their faces; difficult to tell whether because of anger or sadness.

These outbursts frequently happened in my presence. I'd like to think it was because they both felt comfortable with me as a counselor, consequently unafraid of any embarrassment. They displayed openly without ramifications. I acted as a referee; they trusted that neither would hurt the other while in my presence. Hence, the recourse for free-for-all emotional warfare.

Family debates were not always a part of their relationship. Like the ones I witnessed, Raging arguments did not frequently happen, if at all before Brian's present circumstance. Brian's anger toward Sherri was an ancillary occurrence; he was furious at losing his independence. He had to count on Sherri for daily assistance and menial chores. His worst fears were to be obliged to another person. The situation engendered his anger, but it was directed to the person closest to him, as is the case quite often in comparable circumstances.

Sherri piped in again. "Sometimes, when I try to be helpful to him, he gets ugly and swears at me like it's my fault. Why do you get mad at me?" she addressed Brian directly. She stood straight in front of him, glaring with profoundly penetrating but angry eyes.

"I don't know," he said. He wasn't looking directly at Sherri; he looked blankly off toward the television which was on. It sounded less like an answer and more like avoidance. He was tired and did not want more drama. He continued. "I guess it's because I feel like a burden to you… and when you do things for me, it just confirms that feeling…..And I don't like that feeling. I resent being taken care of, and you know that, but do it anyway."

As a referee, I felt obliged to defuse the situation. "I understand that kind of resentment," I said to both of them. They were still fuming. Brian was lying on his stomach with his face in the pillow, and Sherri paced the floor while smoking a cigarette. I had to remind her that smoking in the house with oxygen present was forbidden. She stomped the cigarette out forcefully in a nearby saucer, clearly as a gesture of irritation.

"Sherri takes care of you not because she has to but because she wants to," I said. "She told you you're not a burden, but I guess you can be a challenge at times. She is telling you that you hurt her when you react so furiously at what she does." I don't know why I try to put words in other people's mouths. Sometimes the circumstance requires it.

We had come to an impasse. It became apparent that both Brian and Sherri were simply worn out from their endless quarreling. Without a mandate from me, they each ceased their bellowing at each other. Sherri went outside for another cigarette. Brian rolled over in bed and attempted to fall asleep. Nothing got resolved other than the opportunity to vent, which might have been worth something.

I visited again about a week later. With great trepidation, I entered the house, expecting another round of hassles and hollering. Despite my anticipations, they both appeared reconciled. Resentments surface unexpectedly. I don't think most people hold on to grudges, just waiting for the precise opportunity to unleash them when they know it will cause maximum distress. Instead, they happen. Resentments reside deep inside the soul. A minor provocation lets them loose, and they explode with ferocity and come pouring out without hesitancy or self-control. Grievances have a life of their own. Once we generate them, we continually feed them until they overwhelm us.

Sherri and Brian had been harboring grudges long ago buried in their subconscious. These grudges awakened by the circumstances of a terminal disease. They were as many frustrations about the quality of their own lives as they were grudges directed at the other. Families dealing with a terminal illness and all the consequences of caregiving – the loss of independence, the reality of imminent death, and caregiving challenges – all conspire to generate resentments.

As the spiritual counselor to Brian and Sherri, I was committed to comfort care. Resentments and the attached resilient feelings offered much stress to their relationship. People cling to their grievances as a drowning man clings to a life raft. They feel justified. The obligation to forgive is noticeably absent. One might expect that forgiveness without justification would be possible, even a probability, as a person approaches death. What do they have to lose? Unfortunately, far too many of us go to our graves holding tight to the slightest indignity.

For the remainder of Brian's life with hospice, his relationship with Sherri appeared to border on the verge of a blowup. Brian withdrew from proactive conversation and retreated into his internal thoughts. When he spoke to Sherri, it was reluctantly, responding only with curt answers; yes and no, or I think so. I witnessed no more of Brian's outbursts.

Sherri began to spend less time at home. I would often visit and inquire about her whereabouts. "She's out with some girlfriends," Brian responded. "She needs some time away from me." Brian appeared comfortable with this arrangement, and I had no intentions to inquire further.

When Brian died, Sherri asked me to preside at his memorial service. She provided me with a minimum of information about his life, his likes, and his characteristics. Consequently, I had only marginal material to work with; a few words about his interests in life, some comments about his personality, and some laments that he died too young. Afterward, Sherri indicated the service was "nice," but otherwise, she seemed unimpressed. Satisfied was her demeanor. When she attempted to offer me a check for my "services," and I declined due to hospice policy, she appeared offended. I suggested if she wanted to donate to Hope Hospice, I would pass it on to them. She said that she would not give it to the hospice if the money were not for me. I acted confused and asked if she had a concern about hospice.

"No, not really," she stated. "They did what I suppose they were supposed to do, but I never really like the way they treated Brian."

"How did they treat Brian?"

"Kept changing nurses, even after I asked to keep the same nurse.

"And that made a difference to Brian?"

"It made a difference to me. I just didn't trust hospice after that."

"I'm sorry you feel that way." And then I left her. I felt no need to report this to hospice.

Chapter 18

Ariel's Story - When Death Arrives

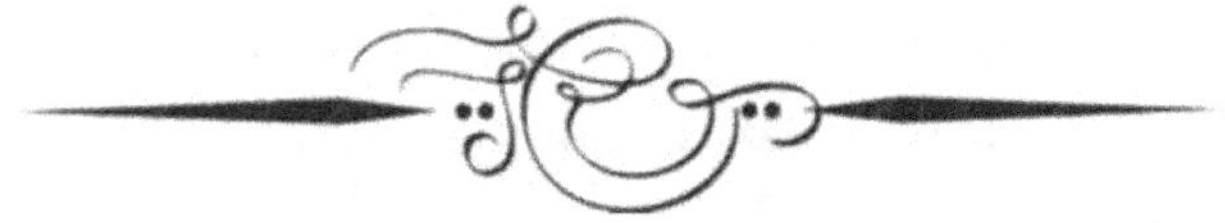

"Life asked death, 'Why do people love me but hate you?' Death responded, Because you are a beautiful lie and I am a painful truth."

- Unknown

The writing was on the wall, the inevitable came, there was a clear recognition; Ariel was in the dying process. It was time to take her home. We knew she would not balk at this; it was never her intention to stay at the hospital.

"Mom," Kimberly tried to awaken her. "Mom, we are taking you home tomorrow morning."

Ariel didn't' answer her but her eyes focused on Kimberly's face and implied clearly that, yes, she understood. it was time to go home.

"We have her on our service" one of the hospice nurses stated who was in the room with us. "We can follow her at home just as well as here in the hospital, maybe better"

A second nurse added, "We can keep her comfortable at home as well as here."

And then a third nurse. "The meds that she is taking can go home with her. There is no interruption in that because we order the same meds through hospice and they will be delivered to your house in the morning. We can get a bed and a table and any other medical equipment ordered today and it will come to your house by tomorrow morning. "Do you have room for a hospital bed? She asked.

"I will have to move some stuff around, but it can go in our bedroom," I told her. "Is that the best place for the bed?" I asked.

"That's up to you. Some people prefer the bed be in the living room because the patient likes to see what's going on at home. Either way, you have to make room for the bed. They will set it up for you, but they can't move any of your furniture. You have to do that."

All these details taken care of by the hospice nurses felt comforting. I usually balk when other people want to do things on my behalf, but at that moment, I appreciated that someone else was taking the responsibility.

Both kids decided to stay overnight in the hospital with Ariel. They encouraged me to go home "You need to get some sleep, dad," they admonished me. I did leave, headed for home, but knew it was not to sleep.

I went into our bedroom and started to dismantle our king-size bed. It had to be removed entirely, the mattress, the frame, and the headboard. It was a major challenge, but I was determined to complete this task tonight. When completely disassembled, I carried each part separately and stored them in the garage. Seeing no bed in the house, the same bed that Ariel and I shared for so many years, conjured up a few tears. It hit me hard that things have changed and will change more before this experience is over. That night what sleep I got was in the spare bedroom. It just didn't feel right.

Early the next morning, just as I was leaving for the hospital, a truck pulled into our driveway blocking my exit to the street.

"Where do you want the bed?" the driver queried.

"It goes in our bedroom," I told him. "It's right inside that door." I pointed to the door at the back of the garage.

The driver had the bed inside and set up in a matter of minutes. It looked strange. A bed with railings and wires attached to it connected to a remote control. It could move up and down, raise or lower the head or feet, and had an attached table; everything imaginable that one would need for an extended time in bed. It was on wheels that could be locked or unlocked depending on where it needed to be placed at any one time. It was a hospital bed and I could not help feeling we were not really leaving the hospital. Emotionally it was difficult to accept.

I returned to the hospital. I told the kids and one of the hospice nurses that the bed had arrived and was assembled. "I guess we can order the ambulance," the nurse told me. "Let me finish the discharge papers and then I will call them."

"Can we ride in the ambulance with mom?" the kids asked

"Absolutely." She responded. They sounded almost like they were anticipating a carnival ride.

"It will be a couple of hours before she is discharged," the nurse reminded us. "Her doctor has to sign off and orders need to be made for continuing medication."

When the doctor showed up, he was less than cooperative.

"Why do you want to take her home?" he asked. By the tone of his voice, I could tell he didn't approve. "She can get better care here. The PET tests the oncologist wants to do can be done here. She can get nursing care here. I think it would be better for her to stay here in the hospital where we can keep an eye on her and administer her medications properly." We knew this doctor was not a big fan of hospice care. Some doctors feel threatened by palliative care procedures; believing it is not real medicine because the care can be given at home. We were prepared for his reluctance.

Kimberly opened the conversation. "Mom wants to be home," she insisted. "She only likes working at the hospital but has real adversity to being in the hospital. We have all considered our options and we all agreed that going home was best for her. Even mom agreed," Kimberly added.

The hospice nurse felt she needed to interject. "All her meds can be ordered through us and we will have our nurse administer them at home."

Rebecca had an opinion as well, probably well-rehearsed just for this occasion. "Mom does not have much time left as best as we can figure and we want her to be where she is most comfortable. Home is where she wants to be and where she will be most comfortable. We can arrange for extra duty caretakers to be present if we are not able to do it all ourselves." She told this to the doctor with a certain amount of authority in her voice,

The three of us, plus the hospice nurse and Mom stopped talking altogether and just stared at the doctor. He realized he had met his match.

"Okay," he eventually said. "I need some time to complete the discharge papers." He left the room and that seemed to settle it. Mom was going home.

The ambulance backed into the driveway. I watched as the driver carefully moved the van as close as possible to the garage door. He asked me if I was ready for Ariel to come inside.

"I think so," I replied. "As ready as I can be."

Kimberly and Rebecca jumped out of back having ridden in the ambulance home. Carol, a friend of Ariel's was also standing by the garage door next to me.

"Wait a minute," Rebecca yelled. "Wait until we get inside." Both of them. along with Carol, went into the house through the garage door.

I turned to the ambulance driver. "I guess we are ready now," I told him.

As the rear door opened further, I saw Ariel sitting upright on the gurney. She spied me. She had the biggest smile on her face. She said nothing, just stared at me. I just about wet my pants when I looked at her. Here I was feeling sorry for myself, thinking that Ariel was coming home to die and I would be left alone. All our plans for retirement down the toilet. I felt so bad; bad about my selfish feelings and bad about Ariel coming home to die. either way, life was not pleasant at that moment.

Ariel, on the other hand, was like a light shining in the darkness. A radiant smile on her face, indicating how happy she was to know she was going home as if she had not a care in the world. If she could speak to me, I am sure she would say, "What are you worrying about? Don't be such a wimp. I am home where I belong. I'll take care of you"

Carol was a nurse who worked with Ariel at the hospital. They had been friends beyond just a working relationship. It was Carol's daughter, who was the head nurse on the medical floor where Ariel was hospitalized. Carol learned about Ariel's situation from her daughter.

Carol was aware of Ariel's resistance to being a patient in the hospital. Both of them had talked at length over the years about how they loved working at the hospital but pleaded with their respected husbands not to ever admit them to a hospital.

Carol had visited with Ariel one afternoon at the hospital to commensurate with her over her having to be in the hospital. Surely, she was there to offer comfort and assistance as well. While there, however, Carol cornered me and insisted that she wanted to be at our house when Ariel was sent home. I suggested to her that perhaps Ariel might never come home. She was a lot more positive than I and continued to assert that she wanted to be present to us at home as well as at the hospital. She was most persistent and I thanked her but without any real understanding of how she might help other than to visit occasionally.

Carol was there to meet us when Ariel got out of the ambulance at home. She never left again until five hours after Ariel's death.

Carol was at Ariel's side twenty-four seven. One time she left to go to the bathroom, that's all I can remember. She fed her, she changed her, she was at Ariel's side when she unconsciously tried to get out of bed. She held her hand and calmed her with soothing words of understanding. When Ariel's lips got too dry from breathing through her mouth, Carol gently moistened her lips with a sponge. The few times when Ariel awoke and was somewhat lucid, but scared, Carol reassured her all was well and patted her head until she relaxed or fell asleep.

"I want to be here all the time, and I mean all the time," Carol insisted

"How can you do that. You have your own family?" I responded

"I can do it, don't worry. I will do it not because I have to but because I want to. I love Ariel."

About every hour, I kept asking her, "How can you do this?" and the answerer was always the same, "I can do it because I want to."

"But you are here twenty-four hours a day. Don't you need to sleep?" I think I was testing her. I couldn't believe her stamina. I knew she wanted to be present for Ariel, but twenty-four/seven, that sounded incredible.

"Just leave me be," Carol reiterated each time I questioned her persistence or her commitment, "This is where I want to be right now."

Not that I objected. It was her endurance I couldn't fathom; her ability to remain present and alert at all times, never leaving Ariel's side. She brought out the guilt I was burying. I had shoved deep down inside my culpability at not taking full responsibility myself for Ariel's care and pawned it off onto other people, onto Carol and the kids.

I had no assurance that Ariel would die in the next hour, or the next day or the next week; only that a preachment had been made that her death was imminent according to the judgment of the medical community. She might be gone at any moment or hang on for a considerable time. It was the ambivalence of the circumstance that bothered me. Another crapshoot

Over the next twenty-four hours. Ariel fluctuated between cognition and stupor. Sometimes she responded briefly when addressed by one of us directly. Otherwise, she remained inert

"Mom, do you need anything?" Kimberly asked her speaking solely and directly to her.

"Is that you Kimberly?" she responded equally slowly. "What are you here for?" Her words were labored and often not related to the question

Marie, our oldest granddaughter sat on the bed and said nothing. "Is that you Marie?" asked Ariel? How did she know it was Marie? We were astonished sometimes by her recognition powers. When she awoke, she looked around the room to see who was present but we did not know if she recognized any of us.

Still other times she reacted with agitation; trying desperately to get out of bed. There was a distinct expression of pain on her face, her arms flailed as if fighting with someone. She reached out and grabbed the handrails of the bed and clutched them securely. We had a difficult time releasing her hand grips on those rails when she was agitated. Carol proved indispensable at times like this. She remained cool and collected encouraging Ariel to remain calm and assured her she was fine. Ariel unfailingly responded positively to Carol's gentle touch and soothing words. She worked miracles.

Most times she appeared to be sleeping. She might have just been rendered unconscious by the pain relief medicines administered and monitored by the hospice's nurses. I was never sure which. The drugs were in control. Although they kept her peaceful, they also induced a comatose stage that sometimes felt like she had stopped breathing and died.

People came and went. My neighbor who worked for another hospice stopped by. Other friends occasionally came for a few minutes, some brought food. The hospice medical director came to the house. Everybody who visited asked, "If there is anything we can do, just ask." Words of empathy were always offered by not always acknowledged by me.

During the afternoon my granddaughters, Marie and Sophia, climbed up on the bed with Ariel with no prompting from anybody. My first reaction was to ask them to get down, but then I thought, what better way for her to die than having her grandchildren by her side. They seemed comfortable sitting there. They expressed no anxieties, almost as if they understood the circumstance and thought it all-natural, even to a kid. Perhaps they were not aware of her imminent death. They asked no questions. Never looked confused

I remember learning early in my pastoral counselor training that it was unwise to answer questions that young children are not asking regarding the meaning of death. Better to allow them to witness the experience and wait until their curiosity emerges. When they are ready, they will formulate their questions using language appropriate to their age level, and only when that is done are they susceptible to explanations by adults.

Time appeared as a blur during the two days Ariel was at home. I was told by my kids that friends came, stayed a while, and then left without my mindfulness. I can only hope I was cordial and receptive; I just don't remember. Neighbors brought food; I didn't eat. I picked at the casserole my neighbor brought in, I can not remember what kind of casserole it was. I lost my taste, didn't want to eat.

I walked into the bedroom where Ariel lay with Carol at her side and then left almost immediately. If Carol said she was alright at the time, I felt I wanted to leave. I found staring at her without her response to be difficult and demeaning. Under my breath, I prayed for a quick death. Guilt overwhelmed me. I urged her to "let go." I knew she was hurting, I was hurting, and I wanted it to end. "Please Ariel, let go, just let go"

I walked outside, wandered around the backyard, inspected the garden without really seeing it, and pretended to pull weeds. Anything to divert my thoughts even if just for a moment.

While I was standing by the garden not looking at it, one of the hospice nurses approached me. We stood regarding each other for an awkward moment, as if sizing each other up upon first meeting. Suddenly she reached out and grabbed me by my shoulders and proceeded to draw me into a hug, wrapping her arms around me

"I think she is active," she told me. "She is about to die soon. She is passing away quickly." I exploded in tears, crying uncontrollably. "Do you want to come inside now?" she continued.

I didn't answer. I followed her toward the house and entered the bedroom where Ariel lay. She was motionless, not breathing. I stared at her.

Carol whispered to me, "She has passed." We both cried. I gazed at her. She looked beautiful as usual. Both my grandchildren sat on the bed, not crying, but holding grandma's hand. Kimberly and Rebecca stood nearby holding each other. They slowly walked toward me and we together held each other, not speaking nor crying anymore. Ariel lay there as if resting after a long day at work.

I bent over and kissed her on the lips, long and hard like I always had, and then my daughters did the same. In between sobs I heard each daughter say directly to Ariel, "Goodbye Mom, I will miss you very much. I love you."

We all stood silently for a few moments, looking at Ariel then looking at each other, and again back at Ariel. "If you are sure you are ready to let her go, I can call the funeral home," one of the hospice nurses said. "Is there anyone else you want to come to say goodbye?"

It suddenly felt stifling in the room. I needed air. I stared at Ariel again and then suddenly departed. I went into the garage. It felt like a train had just plowed into me and knocked all the life out of me. I grabbed a wrench that was lying on the workbench and threw it with all my might out the garage door and hit the front of my car parked in the driveway. It crashed and left a dent. It made no difference then; I was just so angry.

Standing by the edge of the driveway, I felt tears well up in my eyes. Soon they came flowing forth and running freely down my cheeks. I erupted in sobs, uncontrollably bawling. The front of my shirt was soaked.

"No, this can't be," I yelled at the top of my lungs not addressing anyone in particular. I was angry; angry at God, angry that God took Ariel, angry that all our plans now had to be changed, angry that she "decided" to die and leave me alone, angry that I felt selfish and thinking only about myself.

Kimberly and Rebecca soon appeared in the garage. The funeral van arrived after about a half-hour. Someone had called them for me. I was okay with that. I said goodbye again to Ariel, while she lay on a gurney. They placed her in the van. The van drove away with her. She was gone.

The kids brought me back inside to the living room. The grandchildren, Marie and Sophia sat on the couch watching cartoons on the television. Carol had made them each a peanut butter and jelly sandwich. I felt no need to console them; they appeared content. I had no idea what they were thinking but thought it best to not ask now.

"Dad, you need to call Uncle Michael and let him know," Kimberly urged me. Ariel's brother, Michael, lived on Cape Cod. I had a flashback. Michael had some unresolved difficulties with how I cared for Ariel while she was sick. I did not want to confront him now.

"Should I call the Shagorys?" she asked.

"Yes, please do," I responded. That would be helpful."

People began to leave the house shortly after that and always with a hug and some words of condolence. "If there is anything we can do Please call," or "I am so sorry for your lose," or "I will keep in touch soon." I didn't pay much attention. The shock of her death was beginning to set in. I was trying to deny it. I considered how I was going to move on.

Chapter 19

Out of Control

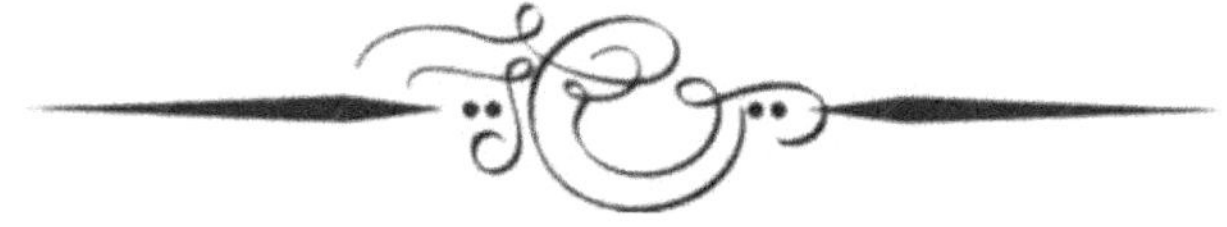

"It is what it is. Isn't that how these things always go?
They are what they are. We just get to cope."

- Mira Grant

Some days you get the bear, and some days the bear gets you. Certain hospice patients were enigmas to me, individuals, who despite suffering from a terminal disease and qualifying for hospice services, with whom I could not make meaningful contact. They or I remained aloof to the relationship for various reasons - barriers between personalities or differences in expectations. Who knows for sure? I felt I was not skilled enough to support the particular patient at that place and at that time. I lacked the specific skills necessary. I failed to connect. I was not a chaplain for them.

Not every patient of hospice is a success story, if by success one means made comfortable during their illness. Sometimes despite our best efforts to provide support for the terminally ill, we fail miserably. This particular patient was an enigma from the beginning. Perhaps he should not have been accepted into the hospice program. But because he was accepted, I felt a commitment to be his chaplain. Unfortunately, that made little impression on him.

Mike's Story

Michael came on our service one day in late November. I remember trying to find the physical address given on his admission form. It was a dreary, cloudy day and beginning to get cold. November is never a pleasant month in Texas, not one about which the chamber of commerce brags. I was not able to see the house's number because of a constant drizzle.

After wandering around in the neighborhood where the GPS indicated Michael lived, I discovered a lone trailer home without any address marker. By process of elimination, since the number next door on one side was a number higher and the other side a number lower, I figured this must be the location. It was between the two numbered houses.

I parked in the dirt alongside the trailer, got out of the car, and with my laptop computer in hand, I approached the front door. There was no doorbell visible but a sign that read "beware of dog." I knocked loudly with my fist. Immediately loud barking came from inside the house. My first reaction was flight; I wanted to run back to the car and get the hell out of there. Visions of raging guard dogs with sharp fangs flashed through my mind. Something about trailers and dogs spooked me. I encountered large and vicious dogs almost exclusively at these locations. But I didn't run. I just froze. Eventually, I heard a voice coming from inside.

"Come on in," the voice stated. "The dogs are harmless, just noisemakers."

I yelled back loud enough to be heard inside the house, "That's what they all say."

"No, it's okay," the voice yelled back. "Come in. The dogs are really friendly. I can't get to the door. I am in bed."

Once hospice admits a patient into the program, each of the assigned staff – nurse, social worker, and chaplain - has a certain number of days to contact the patient. Today was the last day. I needed to complete the initial assessment now.

"Okay," I yelled through the door once again. "I'm coming in. I need the dogs secured." I didn't hear any reply. I took my chances and slowly opened the door. Inside I was accosted by two large dogs of different breeds, both of which started licking my hand and wagging their tails furiously. Friendly? They were more than pleasant; they wouldn't leave my side and followed each step I took. They stayed by my feet as if I were their long-lost owner about to feed them.

It was dark inside. I noticed the shades were pulled down. Michael was sitting on a bed near a window. Adjacent to the bed was a table. On the table were scattered bits of cookies, an empty beer can or two, and an ashtray was overflowing with cigarette butts. Next to the table was an oxygen machine. Michael had the oxygen tube in his nose.

I remember reading in the admitting nurse's notes that Michael's home was not his home, but the home of some friend who felt sorry for him and invited him to stay with her.

"You Michal?" I asked.

"Yep"

I introduced myself as the hospice chaplain. I immediately added, "You can't smoke with oxygen in the house. You know that, don't you?

"Yeah, Yeah, your nurse has been all over me about that."

I had the feeling that he would oblige me while I was there, but the moment I left, he'd light up regardless.

"You can blow yourself up," I told him. "One spark, and you won't need hospice; you'll need an undertaker."

No response from Michael. I think he previously got the same lecture from our nurse who had visited the day before.

I asked Michael if this was his trailer.

"No, it belongs to Susan," he told me

"How do you know Susan?"

"Just a friend," he responded. "She lets me stay here."

Just at that moment, I heard a car drive up to the side of the trailer. After a few moments, a young woman came inside.

"Who are you?" she asked me.

" I'm a chaplain from hospice here to visit Michael, our patient. Michael tells me you let him stay here with you," I said. "Have you known him for a long time?"

"No, He's just a friend of a friend who hangs around here a lot." She then turned to Michael, "You don't have a permanent place to stay around here, do you, Michael?" she asked him.

Michael mumbled something unintelligible.

"I didn't want him hanging around with his druggy friends, she told me. "Especially when he is so sick, so I said he could stay here if he wanted to."

Michael appeared utterly disheveled. His clothes were dirty, His hair was straggly and hung over his eyes, He kept trying to push it away, but it fell back in his face. I am not a judgmental person, but I immediately had thoughts that Michael was a drug user and homeless. Susan felt sorry for him and, being a caring person or perhaps a drug-using cohort, invited him to be there where it was safe for both of them to use if they pleased.

Michael, perhaps sensing what I was thinking, interrupted my thoughts. "She lets me shack out here cause I got no other place to stay, that's all. I ain't using stuff now, not while I am here," he insisted.

Not all our patients live with adequate accommodations. Some have few resources and live in trailers or low rent-subsidized apartments. Many exist on the edge of collapse, but I had yet to discover a patient living in such squalor as Michael. He claimed he had no immediate family, at least none that he would admit. There was no family caretaker. He acknowledged Susan as a "friend" but didn't volunteer to talk about becoming friends. She offered a place for Mike to hang out, so he took it.

He had no explanation for where he lived before now. I didn't ask.

Mike felt no pain; I suspect because he had been on drugs and was probably still using even now or living with the effects of his last drug shoot-up. I was afraid to ask. By the end of this initial visit, I was beginning to like Mike. He was pleasant, didn't whine or complain about his circumstances, and always agreed to whatever conditions we placed on him – no smoking with oxygen in place, no drugs other than those we prescribed, and no sharing of the medicines we prescribed with his friends. Mike responded positively to our mandates. But I never could tell if he was being genuine or telling me a fictional story. That was my opinion for the first weeks.

"If I smoke, I go outside." He assured me. "I hide the drugs you give me. I aint using any other drugs, no more, I ain't." He was so compliant that he fooled all three of his hospice workers, the nurse, the social worker, and me.

Over the next few weeks, there were no changes in Mike's circumstance. He remained at the home of his friend Susan and was usually on his bed each time I stopped by. I tried to call before arriving but didn't connect by phone.

"Mike, what is the matter with your phone?" I asked on one visit

"Nothing," he replied. "Why?"

"I call and call, and no answer. Sometimes it tells me the phone number is no longer available."

He reached for his phone on the table next to him, pushed a few of its buttons, and declared, "It's dead. I forget to charge it."

"You got to keep it working. If you need us or we need you, we have to have a working phone."

No response.

On one visit not long after the lecture he got about sharing drugs with friends, he notified us that he had run out of medicines. We visited Mike in pairs because we learned his neighborhood was infested with drug users and might not be the safest place for a single nurse or social worker to be wandering through alone. I was the only male on the team, so the staff tagged me always to accompany the females.

"Mike, your pills are gone for this period, and it's too early to renew your prescription. Where did they all go?" Most of Mike's prescriptions were for controlled drugs.

He had no answer. We suspected that he was either overdosing or sharing with friends. We learned that he had previously been on probation for drug use. When confronted with this evidence, he swore up and down that he no longer abused drugs. He emphatically stated that he stopped that after learning he had COPD.

He had a demeanor of pity about him and appeared so pathetic that I found it difficult to deny him hospice services. Our standard policy is to immediately dismiss a patient who we can demonstrate abusing the medications we provide. Mike presented me with a dilemma. Hospice policy dictates that we provide comfort care to those meeting the hospice criteria. Hospice staff makes all attempts to be as empathic as possible, not denying relief to those in pain. Michael was clearly in pain but at the same time out of compliance with hospice policy. What to do about Mike?

One day I went to visit Michael and he was gone. His trailer was empty except for the dogs. I tried calling his phone, but no response.

"Well, I thought, this solves the dilemma on drug abuse for hospice. If Mike took off, it's not our responsibility to go looking for him." I felt relief. I no longer had to decide about his continuing on our service. He decided for us. Not so quick, however.

Exactly one week later, the nurse got a phone message from Michael. He offered apologies and expressed sorrow. He claimed he had been kicked out of Susan's trailer because her boyfriend objected to his presence, perhaps thinking him a competitor or interloper. Mike left an address nearby where he could we could find him.

The next day I showed up at that address. It was a dilapidated house just off the side of the road with a damaged car parked in the dirt driveway. I knocked on the front door, and while I was waiting, I heard loud voices coming from inside. I heard two people screaming at each other, a man and a woman, each calling the other the vilest of names. Suddenly there was silence. The screaming ceased, and a woman came to the door. Politely and calmly, she inquired, "What do you want?'

"I'm looking for Mike," I told her

"He's out back." She pointed to a shed at the back of the yard. I told her I was from hospice and he was a patient of ours,

"Go on back," she said. "Good luck, he's a beauty."

A tall man appeared at the door, disheveled and quite clearly influenced by some sort of drug. He stared at me.

"This is my husband, "she said. "He's a friend of Mikes." It confirmed for me that Mike also was still doing drugs. Guilty by association. He was still staring at me as I moved toward the shed in the backyard.

The shed was about twenty by twenty with no windows, just a plywood door. Inside, there was a hole in the wall where a window air conditioner was attached and running full force. Still, it was stifling inside.

I never knew precisely the age of Michael. His appearance was so unkempt. I found him to be a paradox; his emaciated face gave the impression of early-onset aging, but the rest of his body, though extremely slight, and withered gave the appearance of a younger man.

Inside were assortments of faded Playboy centerfolds plastered on the walls along with a couple of dozen menacing knives of different sizes and shapes hanging from hooks or mounted on plywood. One's first impression was this is the den of a lunatic killer or madman. Peter, back away as fast as you can. But Michael never gave off frightening vibes. Instead, he proved to be a most gentle person. He associated with bad company and unsuspectingly got caught up in a web of bad decisions leading to dire consequences.

I could not condone Michael's actions, but neither could I condemn him. I had to focus on the person with a terminal disease. Try as I might, I could not ignore my feelings of compassion for a man whose life focus was solely upon trying to feel good, without the insipid and constant pain of his disease. He didn't ask for this diagnosis. It was not a result of his lifestyle; drug use was probably not a cause of his COPD. It just happened, and he deserved what comfort hospice therapy could provide. For the time being, we continued to be his "caretaker" and provided pain relief despite our awareness of his abuse of the drugs and despite his resistance to suggested changes in lifestyle with which we consistently bombarded him. But we reached Michael too late.

The hospice program cannot continue to exist without strict adherence to policy. The hospice staff decided that we could no longer provide the service, knowing that Mike either refused to abide by regulations or was simply no longer able to do so. Michel left our program, never to be heard from again. One of my greatest regrets as a hospice chaplain.

Chapter 20

Ariel's Story -Moving On

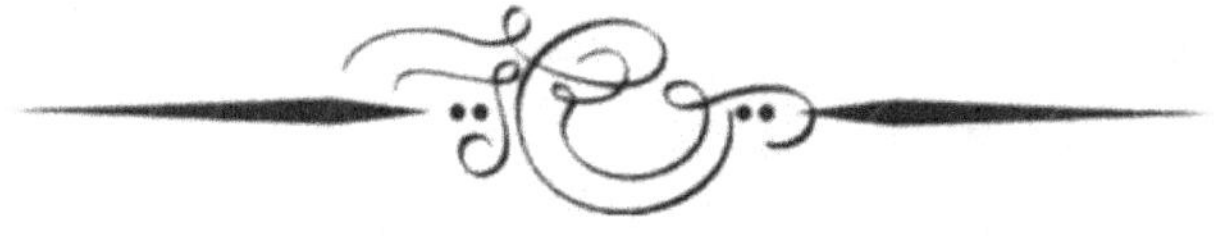

"Pain makes you stronger, tears make you braver, and heartbreak makes you wiser, so thank the past for a better future."

- Unknown

"All deaths are sudden no matter how gradual the dying may be."

- Michael McDowell

"How are you feeling now about Ariel's death?" A close friend and fellow pastor asked me one day shortly after she passed.

I don't know how I feel," I told him. "I am sure I have some feelings; I just can't sort them out yet, probably because there are so many feelings coming so fast."

The numbness had not worn off. The severity of the experience and the mish-mash of feelings overwhelmed me that I thanked people for their concerns but probably never really heard their concerns. Neighbors left casseroles in my kitchen, invitations were forthcoming for dinners out with friends, and requests that I should attend support groups ("They help you adjust") were plentiful those first few weeks following Ariel's death. My feelings still felt too raw to allow me to share much with others. I hung back and stayed to myself. The numbness had not yet worn thin enough to venture out.

The hospice Ariel worked for held a brief memorial service in the facility chapel. Kimberly and I decided to attend. Coworkers shared accolades about Ariel; memories each had about things she had done or left undone, her personality, commitment to hospice, empathy toward patients, and compliments about her character. I was duly impressed by their sincerity.

As I left the facility, I noticed a flower garden adjacent to the hospice office front door. It immediately struck me as a perfect place to spread some of Ariel's ashes when they returned. I did so with the blessing of the Hospice personal.

I looked again at the garden. I pointed to a particular bush and asked, "What do you call those big red flowers that look like roses?" I don't know," she answered. "They look like roses to me, but I know they are not roses. Why do you ask?"

"Ariel's favorite flower is the red rose," I told her." Perhaps I can plant a rose bush right here after we bury her ashes; a red rose bush. What do you think?"

"Don't know about protocol," the nurse responded, but my feelings are let's do it and worry about forgiveness later."

"Can I get in touch with you when I receive her ashes back?" I asked.

Please do", she responded. I left feeling some hopefulness for the first since her death.

The beauty of cremation is that it provides for a memorial service. The family plans the memorial service rather than the funeral director. No law says you need to have a memorial service within a particular time frame that suits the undertaker. Memorial services can occur wherever and whenever the family chooses – in a meadow among the woods on a sunny afternoon, by the seashore early in the morning, on top of a mountain, in a private home, or a church sanctuary. The family chooses the time and place depending on what they feel is important.

My first concern was my family. I needed to have family present at Ariel's memorial service. The place was secondary in my considerations. As I gave it thought, I choose a small congregational church in our town, a church to which both Ariel and I had some connection and among people we knew. I had a hunch that there would be a sizable crowd who wanted to attend once they knew of the time and place. The church sanctuary seemed sufficient for the number of people I expected to participate.

The minister was a colleague of mine, appropriately sensitive, empathetic, and a friend of Ariel's. He would conduct the service, a celebration of life rather than a service of grief, paying most attention to joyful memories and least attention to heartache and grief. However, neither should be discounted if bereavement is authentic.

During my time as pastor, I had planned dozens and dozens of memorial services for church members and friends. For some reason, however, I approached this service with apprehension. I got the worst feeling that I might be planning a service to which no one would attend. I planned my mother's memorial service a few years previous and was greatly dismayed when only two women showed up. I took it personally. I felt it a slight not only on my mother but on me. People I knew did not find it essential to support me at the time of my mother's demise. It felt like pure rejection. I had buried these feelings, and now, as I planned for Ariel's service, these feelings crept back into my thoughts.

Kimberly remained at home for a week following Ariel's death; I suspect she wanted to be sure I was coping well. I appreciated her attention but also wanted to be alone for a while. We survived together, and together we planned for the memorial service. We agreed on the celebration, the date and time, on food for a reception, on pictures to be shown at the service, and on the "focus" for the service; that it be a celebration of life.

The service proved to be as I imagined. All my family, daughters, some cousins, spouses of brothers, and a whole host of friends of ours were present. I felt assured they would not think of missing this occasion, and they didn't. Not a single nurse who worked with Ariel at Hope Hospice missed this event. During the service, one of the nurses offered a eulogy in which she cited Ariel's ability as a nurse and her commitment to hospice. Also, she had a little fun describing Ariel's propensity for getting lost when visiting patients at home and presented her posthumously with the "Directionally Challenged" award for the year.

My friend Xavier sang some tribute songs for Ariel that I requested. While he was performing, slides of Ariel were posting on a large screen behind him. When a picture of Ariel in a bikini shone brightly above his head, people began to snicker and giggle. Poor Xavier thought they were laughing at his singing. I assured him later that this was not the case.

Following the memorial service, we gathered in the fellowship hall for a shared meal together. Various people took advantage of the occasion to offer tributes and memories, both serious and laughable to Ariel. I am sure that those present genuinely wanted to express concern, but my feelings remained numb. It was as if I were still in a dream and had not yet woken up. I remember the rest of the afternoon because I was concerned that people were not getting enough food, that perhaps they didn't like the catered food available. They were eating it, that's for sure, and I could see that, but they did so only out of empathy for me. How did I feel about their empathy? I found it difficult to accept. I do not remember thinking it was ingenious, but rather that I didn't deserve it, didn't want it, didn't find it comforting. Empathy made me feel uncomfortable, as if something was happening to me that I could not control by myself.

Afterward, I puzzled over my reaction to the empathy I felt from friends. What bothered me? Was I responding "unempathetically" toward people who are sincerely attempting to be concerned, be sympathetic at Ariel's death, the loss of my wife?

After considerable thought and reflection, I came to the following conclusion. Many people, including myself, do not want to feel weak or incapable. I pride myself on feeling sufficient, independent. When people express empathy towards me, as they did on the occasion of Ariel's death, I felt vulnerable. I saw myself as less potent than usual and less powerful than others. It felt like pity, and pity is an emotion I understand that designates a person less than fully human. The more empathy received, the more tendency to feel pity.

Now, this is simply an explanation for my feeling less than enthusiastic towards receiving empathy. I do not let it get in the way of my relationship with those who offer that empathy—just the opposite. I fully understand and appreciate that they show care and concern, and I am sure that I will continue to try to be an empathic person in the future.

The biggest drawback for me at the time of Ariel's death was that I lived in a community where I failed to make friends. Like many other people, especially men, professional people mainly, I had many people I associated with but none of whom I counted as friends. I hesitated to get emotionally close to others. Getting close meant sharing feelings, thoughts, wishes, dreads, and more, and getting close meant sharing yourself and your flaws with someone else who accepts you. Outside of Ariel, none in my life met that criteria. I did not feel lonely; instead, I felt aloof from potential friends. I kept them at a distance.

Parting Thoughts

Although I appreciated the messages, the thoughts, the emails from friends saying "sorry for your loss," they still came as stinging reminders of what has just happened. I was in denial and didn't want to face what had happened continually. I closed myself off; I didn't want to talk about it. I internalized what pain I was feeling, stuffed it down, hoping it might just go away. I kept everything inside and tried not to show how messed up I was, how badly I was handling this death, trying to build an emotional dungeon where I could store away the terrible feelings, some of which were feelings of guilt. The guilt was at times overwhelming; that I should have done things differently continued to haunt me. When people die, we always feel guilty about; things we wished we had done or not done. Yes, it does feel awful to be angry at someone for dying, but when I examined my anger, I concluded that I was not mad at a person for dying, but angry because they have died.

Sometimes when I felt myself thinking back at how I acted during Ariel's long illness, I feel shame. I feel shame that I had feelings of anger at her for being sick. Indeed, there were feelings of guilt; the guilt I felt that I had not done enough, that I could have done more, that I should have done more, but I also realized that the "couldof, shouldof, wouldof" feelings were normal and I would survive despite these feelings. I stopped punishing myself for those feelings.

What I had difficulty moving past was the guilt I felt knowing that there were times during her sickness when I just felt angry; angry at her for being sick, angry at God for allowing this to happen to her, and more importantly, anger at anybody and anything that disrupted my plans for the future that included the death of Ariel. While Ariel lay dying, even before her last breath when I was supposed to be feeling empathy, I acknowledge that I was hoping for a quick death, not just to alleviate her suffering but mine as well. My anger seemed to be stronger than my grief. I learned somewhere that anger could be your body's reaction to a threat. The threat can be real or perceived. There is nothing more threatening than death. Anger is your body's natural reaction to the threat of death.

Feeling numb was the overriding feeling I experienced. A person may expect emotional numbness after death; that's easy to tell another person, but when it's yourself, the feeling is unexplainable. You just feel numb. Rationally I knew of ways to heal emotional numbness, but I was not yet ready to go there, to be rational. I knew I could never go back to "normal," that will not happen. There is no time limit to grief, and remembrances can leave you reeling. Still, the intensity of grief tends to lessen with time. But over time, I felt stronger, and with strength, I was able to move on eventually. That's where people have to go, and that's where I am headed.

One last thought. About four or five years before Ariel passed. I planted a Rosebush in our front year. For five years, the bush just sat there, neither growing nor dying, just sitting there. The year following Ariel's passing, we had sufficient rains and clear, cool weather one spring. The rose bush, like magic, grew up to three feet in height over a brief period and bloomed profusely with large red roses. Why Now, I wondered.